Desserts for Diabetics

Desserts for Diabetics

OVER 200 RECIPES FOR DELICIOUS TRADITIONAL DESSERTS ADAPTED FOR DIABETIC DIETS

Mabel Cavaiani, R.D.,
with Anne Blocker, R.D., L.D.

FOREWORD BY DR. GARY D. GILMORE

A PERIGEE BOOK

A Perigee Book
Published by The Berkley Publishing Group
A division of Penguin Putnam Inc.
375 Hudson Street
New York, New York 10014

First Perigee edition published 1992
Revised Perigee edition: October 2002

Visit our website at www. penguinputnam.com

Library of Congress Cataloging-in-Publication Data

Cavaiani, Mabel.
Desserts for diabetics : 125 recipes for delicious traditional
desserts adapted for diabetic diets / Mabel Cavaiani, with
Anne Blocker ; foreword by Dr. Gary D. Gilmore.
p. cm.
Previously published: New York : Perigee Books, 1992.
Includes index.
ISBN 0-399-52817-2
1. Diabetes—Diet therapy—Recipes. 2. Desserts. I. Blocker,
Anne Kriener. II. Title.
RC662 .C37 2002
641.5'6314—dc21   2002025245

Printed in the United States of America

20 19 18 17

*In loving memory of Pauline Bever, a true southern lady,
and for her daughters, Mabel Frances Gunsallus, Mary Boineau,
Mildred "Cracker" Holton, and Margaret "Monk" Sellers. We
have been so much a part of each other's lives for so long that I feel
like one of the family.*

and

*In loving memory of Mabel Cavaiani, who passed away during
the revision of this book. Mabel was a true inspiration and
mentor to her friends, colleagues, and clients. Her own personal
experience with diabetes and her love of cooking have helped
thousands of people enjoy great-tasting food as part of their
diabetes self-management. She was indeed a great lady who
touched the lives of all those she met.*

Contents

Acknowledgments

WE WOULD LIKE to thank the many people whose collaboration and friendship have helped us with this book. We especially thank all the people living with diabetes who know that eating is still one of life's greatest pleasures.

Mabel thanks the following people for their encouragement and professional help in developing and writing this book:

Mabel Frances Gunsallus, M.S., R.D., of Miami, with whom I have discussed this, as well as other books I have written, in great detail.

Edith Robinson, M.S., R.D., of Decatur, Georgia, who first encouraged me to write cookbooks for modified diets.

Muriel Urbashich, R.D., of Hometown, Illinois, with whom I have written several books. Her encouragement and professional information have been a great boon to me.

Patti Dillon, M.S., Fayette County (Iowa) Extension Office home economist, whose encouragement and professional information helped make this book a reality.

Kathy Steege, manager, and Judy Mohlis, assistant, Fayette County Extension Office, whose capable computerized nutritive analysis of the recipes furnished information of vital importance to all who use this book.

Vera and Aulden Wilson, of Wadena, Iowa, who tested and discussed many of the recipes.

Frances Nielsen, of Oak Lawn, Illinois, who taught me so much of what I know about food and food preparation.

Diane Daab, of Holland, Michigan, whose handling of her daughter Anna's diabetes is an inspiration to me.

And last but not least, my late husband, Charles Cavaiani, and my sister, Shirley Sniffin. Their patience and support helped make this book possible.

Anne thanks the following people for their assistance, support, encouragement, love, and patience in developing and writing this book:

My husband, Dave, and children, Katie, Marty, and Grace, for their love, patience, and support during the work on this book, for test-tasting recipes and honestly expressing how they tasted, and for keeping me on task regardless of the time of day. I love you all very much.

Rosemary Kriener, my mother, for countless hours of help with computer entry, editing, and sampling foods. But most of all for teaching me how to cook and being patient when I first experimented in the kitchen. I could not have finished this book without your tremendous and unending help. And my dad, Leo Kriener, who taught me at a young age that if you want to eat more than lemon pudding and shredded wheat, you have to learn how to cook. Thank you for being such wonderful parents.

Jeanne Blocker, my mother-in-law, for sharing and modifying recipes and setting up a second test-kitchen when I needed more help cooking. I am so fortunate to have a mother-in-law that is such an awesome cook. And Maurice Blocker, my father-in-law, who tested everything and smiled. Thanks to both of you—I think you're great.

The Upper Iowa District Dietetic Association members for your encouragement, professional knowledge, and answers to my questions along the way, especially M. J. Smith, Julie Cull, Rosemary Behrens, and Sandy Hagen. You are the best friends a dietitian could ever have.

My brother, Joe Kriener, for successfully rescuing recipe files off the computer. You lowered my stress level more than once and helped me keep on track with this project. I am in grateful admiration of your many talents.

Stacy Koehn, who, since age five, has lived life daily with diabetes and never let it keep her from truly living. You are an inspiration to all.

Butch and Jan Franks, dear friends of Mabel, who worked with me on this project when Mabel no longer was able to do so. Mabel was indeed blessed to have had such wonderful friends.

Mabel Cavaiani, for your faith and trust in me to help you with this work and for years of mentoring and support of my dreams. I will treasure our friendship always.

To all the patients and clients I have worked with in the past fifteen years. You have taught me that nutrition and health are really about eating great-tasting foods and being truly satisfied—and working health in along the way.

We would also like to thank the following organizations and publications for background information, resource material, and nutritive information used in this book:

The American Association of Diabetes Educators

The American Diabetes Association

The American Dietetic Association

The American Heart Association

Iowa State University Extension Service

U.S. Department of Agriculture

Diabetes Forecast, the magazine of the American Diabetes Association

Foreword

DIABETES IS AN abnormality in how the body controls levels of blood sugar. The number of those with diabetes is increasing each year, with current levels at approximately 16 million, and up to half are unaware that they have it. It is estimated that 80 percent of those with adult-onset diabetes, or Type 2, are overweight. Overall, persons with diabetes have an increased risk for major complications, such as blindness, cardiovascular disease, kidney failure, and lower-extremity problems requiring amputations. Even with these severe consequences, it has been estimated that up to 85 percent of those with diabetes do not engage in optimal self-care activities, including the planning of appropriate meals. The benefits of adopting a healthier lifestyle have been well documented for those with diabetes, as well as for every person desiring a higher quality of living.

It is important to realize that there is not just one diabetes diet. Overall, the basic recommendation is for a diet low in fats and sugary foods, and with a variety of fresh fruits and vegetables, fish, and lean meats. Additionally, the American Dietetic Association encourages those with diabetes to calculate their total grams of carbohydrate consumed for the control of their blood glucose levels.

A valuable discovery for those with diabetes and their families would be a resource that enables them to live their lives as normally and happily as possible. You will find that this cookbook represents such a resource. In chapter 1, a comprehensive approach to living with diabetes is presented. It becomes clear that change can be adopted gradually. Additionally, family members and friends can reinforce the healthier changes on a daily basis. Subsequent chapters reinforce the importance of properly prepared meals and present clearly described, rather easily prepared recipes.

While remaining true to the original intent and purpose of the book, Anne Blocker has infused some of the newer aspects about "living" with diabetes, to include carbohydrate counting. Throughout the book, Anne also imparts her enthusiasm and energy for holistic living and sharing favorite family recipes with others. Her additions to the original work crafted by Mabel Cavaiani are clear and concise, while conveying helpful updates. Importantly, the reader will find an array of recipes and recommendations. Many of these culinary creations came from suggestions by others, followed by painstaking preparations by Anne, with follow-up testing by her willing family members.

One of the challenges we face as health professionals is attempting to translate what our scientific studies are indicating into appropriate, reasonable, and appealing recommendations for the public. In this carefully crafted book, you will find a resource which addresses that challenge through prudent recipes that actually enliven the taste buds. Bon appétit!

Gary D. Gilmore, M.P.H., Ph.D., C.H.E.S.
Director, Community Health Programs
University of Wisconsin, La Crosse

Introduction

FOOD IS SO much a part of who we are, how we celebrate special occasions and holidays, and how we nourish and nurture our bodies. It is woven into our history and our traditions. Whether it's roasted turkey with candied yams, orange-cranberry relish, and Grandma's pumpkin pie at Thanksgiving or a special cake for a birthday celebration, we like to enjoy great-tasting food. Sometimes, though, health problems cause people to make changes in their food choices. When these changes involve eliminating favorite foods, the decision between health and taste can often be difficult.

We believe that all foods can fit into almost any lifestyle. This may involve a bit of planning, but food should not just be good for us, it should taste delicious. That is why we wrote this book. We believe that people with diabetes need a cookbook of dessert recipes that are scrumptious, traditional, and suitable for their health needs. We also believe the foods should be so appetizing that other members of the family want to eat them too.

So much has changed in the area of diabetes care and management in the past few years. We couldn't have written this book twenty-five years ago, because at that time it was taboo to include sugar in your diet. Well, times have changed and now we know that moderation is the key. No more cheating and feeling bad about having sugar, a sliver of pie, or a gourmet chocolate chip cookie. All foods can fit into a healthy eating plan; it just takes a little creativity and flexibility.

We hope that you find these recipes a welcome addition to your meal planning and that the desserts you make bring joy to your dinner table.

Mabel Cavaiani, R.D.
Wadena, Iowa

Anne Blocker, R.D., L.D.
Waukon, Iowa

CHAPTER 1

Diabetes

As WE HAVE said in other books, this is a cookbook and not a diet manual. However, we don't think it is fair to give you special recipes for persons with diabetes without some discussion of diabetes itself.

First of all, we believe that diabetes is not the end of normal living. So many changes have been made in the past few years in the field of diabetes care to improve health outcomes for people. We now know that people who take care of their diabetes can prevent the complications associated with the disease, including heart disease, vision problems, neuropathy, and stroke. If you have recently discovered you have diabetes, or if you have had it for some time, we recommend you consider the following guidelines.

1. Work with your health care team to learn about diabetes self-management. The more you take charge of managing your diabetes, the better off you will be. Your diabetes team should include a physician, a dietitian, a pharmacist, and a diabetes educator and/or a nurse who specializes in diabetes care. There may be others involved in your care also, such as a podiatrist, a behavior health specialist, and an ophthalmologist, to name a few. You should have contact with members of your health care team annually and follow up on their recommendations for periodic exams and lab tests, including foot and vision screening, hemoglobin A1C testing, nutritional review, and others.

2. Monitor your blood glucose regularly. Learn what high and low blood sugar levels mean for you and how things like activity, food,

alcohol, medication, and illness affect you personally. You are the best person to alert your health care provider if you notice changes in your blood sugar levels that cannot be explained by these variables. It is a good idea to keep a diary of your blood glucose monitoring. Make notes next to your glucose levels of what may have caused any deviations from normal. Many of the new glucometers on the market today will store records for several days that you can print out.

3. Learn how foods affect your blood glucose. For some people this may mean closely following a meal plan. For others, it may mean developing a meal routine that contains the same types of food at each meal. As you work with your dietitian, you will learn how to work all types of foods into your diet.

4. Be active. Physical activity is one of the best ways to promote normal blood glucose levels. In addition, it keeps your muscles strong, burns extra calories, lowers stress, and improves mental health. Check with your health care provider for activities that are best for you. Be sure to get in the habit of checking your feet regularly before and after activities. People with diabetes have to take extra care to keep their feet in good condition.

5. Learn about your medications and take them as prescribed. Keeping track of your blood glucose levels can help you and your physician know how well your medication is working. If you have questions about your medications, always consult your pharmacist and/or physician.

6. Join a diabetes support group and/or subscribe to a diabetes magazine to continue to expand your knowledge about diabetes and to have support available for times when you may need it. Because diabetes is a chronic disease that does not go away, it can be stressful to manage it on a day-to-day basis. Having a group of friends, professionals, and other people with diabetes can be good support.

The American Diabetes Association is an excellent resource for people with diabetes. You can find out more about the American Diabetes Association via the Internet at www.diabetes.org or by writing to them at American Diabetes Association, 1701 North Beauregard Street, Alexandria, VA 22311. Another excellent resource for information about healthy eating is the American Dietetic Association. You can learn more from this organization via the Internet at www.eatright.org or by writing to them at The American Dietetic Association, 216 West Jackson Boulevard, Chicago, IL 60606. To find a support group in your area, contact local hospitals or physicians' clinics.

7. Above all, don't retreat from life. Life is not over. You can have a long and happy and healthy life ahead of you. You can prevent the complications of the disease by learning the strategies of successful dia-

betes self-management. You can go on long trips, get married, have children, be a prominent athlete or famous scientist, or just live and enjoy a happy life. We're sure you can do all these things because many people have done them and told us about it . . . and we know you can too.

CHAPTER 2

Carbohydrate Counting

HAVE YOU HEARD? There is a new way to eat that helps control your blood sugar and allows you to work in all your favorite foods. This new type of meal planning includes carbohydrate counting. We now know that it is the amount of carbohydrate that you eat that affects your blood glucose levels more than the type or source of the carbohydrate food.

In the past, people with diabetes used one primary type of meal-planning tool, called the "Exchange System," for regulating their food intake. While this method of meal planning allows for a well-balanced diet, it can sometimes be confusing and restrictive for people with diabetes who are already struggling to manage the other aspects of the disease. The Exchange System, still used by many people today, is explained in the next chapter.

Carbohydrate counting is another tool people can use to plan their meals to achieve good blood glucose control. Scientific evidence and clinical observation have shown that the carbohydrate in food is the primary nutrient that affects blood glucose levels. For many people, this method of meal planning allows them more variety and flexibility with food, based on their individual blood glucose levels. Your registered dietitian or physician can help you develop a carbohydrate-eating plan that is right for you.

Carbohydrate counting is not a new phenomenon. In fact, this system of meal planning has been used at some medical centers in the United States since 1935 and in Europe for even longer. Within the last four to six years more people with diabetes have been using it on a regular basis.

Here's how carbohydrate counting works: When you eat food or drink certain beverages, your blood glucose level goes up. The amount that your blood glucose rises typically depends on the amounts and types of foods that you eat.

Foods containing mostly carbohydrates will cause your blood glucose level to rise more than foods containing primarily protein and fat. Carbohydrates are found mainly in breads and starches like pasta, rice, cereals, and crackers; fruits, fruit juices; starchy vegetables like corn, peas, and squash; milk and milk products; sweetened carbonated beverages; and desserts and sugars, including jams, jellies, syrups, sugar, and honey. When you know the amount of carbohydrate you are eating, you can predict what your blood glucose response will be.

Large amounts of carbohydrates will typically cause your blood glucose levels to rise more than small amounts will. For example, eating two slices of bread will cause your blood glucose to go up more than eating one slice of bread, and three slices will raise it higher than two.

Liquids, such as juice, milk, or sweetened carbonated beverages, often cause blood glucose to rise faster than solid foods. For example, drinking apple juice will make your blood glucose increase quicker than eating an apple. This happens because solid foods take longer to digest than liquids.

Foods high in protein and fats, such as meats, poultry, fish, butter, oil, margarine, nuts, and seeds, do not seem to raise blood glucose levels as much or as quickly as carbohydrate-containing foods do. For this reason, it is suggested that these foods be eaten in moderation. Moderation would mean 4 to 5 ounces of protein and 3 to 5 servings of fats each day. Your dietitian can help you determine the amounts of carbohydrate, protein, and fat to eat daily.

Carbohydrate information can be found in a variety of places. Carbohydrate is measured in grams. You can use the exchange lists in the next chapter to help you estimate the carbohydrate content of many foods. For example, one bread/starch "exchange" contains 15 grams of carbohydrate. This means that all of the foods listed in the bread/starch group contain about 15 grams of carbohydrate per serving. Foods in the milk group contain 12 grams of carbohydrate, fruits contain 15 grams of carbohydrate, and vegetables (except for the starchy vegetables, which contain 15 grams) contain about 5 grams of carbohydrate per serving.

The nutrition food label on food packages is also a good source of carbohydrate information. The Nutrition Facts panel on the label lists the amount of carbohydrate per serving of the food item. The label also lists information including amount of protein, fat, fiber, and sugar in the food. This information can help you identify differences in the nutritional value of the food items. However, for the purpose of carbohydrate counting, focus on the total grams of carbohydrate per serving. Note that the total grams of sugar per serving of food are included in the total grams of carbohydrate.

In addition to the exchange list and the food label, there are many good books that have nutritional information about foods. These books can be found in bookstores or libraries; often your health care provider can recommend a good reference. Two helpful books listing carbohydrate and other nutritional information about food are *The Complete Book of Food Counts* by Corinne T. Netzer and *The Diabetes Carbohydrate and Fat Gram Guide,* second edition, by Lea Ann Holzmeister.

Your dietitian can help you determine the meal-planning system that will work best for you. If you decide to use the carbohydrate-counting system, you will initially keep track of how much carbohydrate you eat during the day and how it affects your blood glucose levels. Monitoring your intake and blood glucose values will help you and your health care provider decide on any changes you may need to make in your routine—be it food, medication, or exercise.

Keeping track of your daily intake of carbohydrate can be done in one of two ways. Some people prefer to count all the grams of carbohydrate they eat and drink throughout the day. This means that if you need to eat 200 grams of carbohydrate during the day to keep your blood sugar in a normal range, you would ideally divide the 200 grams into three meals and one to three snacks. This would allow you to eat and drink about 45 to 60 grams of carbohydrate at each meal and 15 grams at snack time.

This method takes a bit more diligence, but it is the most precise. If you are working to regulate your medication, it can be the most helpful method.

The other method of carbohydrate counting is to keep track of the number of carbohydrate "choices" you eat and drink during the day. This differs slightly from gram counting in that one carbohydrate choice equals approximately 15 grams of carbohydrate. Therefore, you would count one carbohydrate choice for one serving of bread, an apple, or a small cookie, and instead of the 200-gram allowance, you might plan to eat and drink thirteen carbohydrate choices throughout the day. People who like the exchange system often find this method simpler to use because one starch/bread, fruit, or milk serving equals one carbohydrate choice. While this method tends to be easier for many people to keep track of, it is not as accurate as the gram-counting method mentioned above. It is, however, a simple and easy way to add flexibility to your diet while contributing to good blood glucose control.

As with any method of meal planning, being aware of portion size is important. The recipes in this book provide nutrient information in all three formats: food exchanges, carbohydrate grams, and carbohydrate choices. We hope this book makes it easier for you to achieve good blood glucose control while enjoying all foods—including dessert.

CHAPTER 3

Food Exchanges

BECAUSE THE AMOUNT of carbohydrate (CHO), fat (FAT), and protein (PRO) are significant in the diabetic diet, the American Dietetic Association and the American Diabetes Association have worked together to establish basic food groups to be used as a basis for planning diabetic diets. Your doctor, dietitian, or nutritionist will help you understand the different food groups and how many exchanges (units) from each of the food groups you can have daily.

The starch/bread exchanges are important because they contain most of the carbohydrate in your diet. The amount of carbohydrate is important because carbohydrate forms sugar in the body and people with diabetes have trouble utilizing sugar because they lack insulin (Type 1) or can't utilize the insulin they do have (Type 2) and therefore they need to control the amount of carbohydrate they eat daily.

Meat exchanges are important because they contain protein, which helps maintain muscles and body functions. Vegetable, fruit, meat, and milk exchanges are not used very often in a dessert cookbook, but they are a necessary part of eating healthy. Foods from these groups provide many of the vitamins and minerals needed for good health and should be used according to your exchange allowance.

Fat exchanges are important because they not only add weight but they can contribute to raising the cholesterol level in the blood if the wrong kind (saturated fat) is used too frequently.

The following table lists the various exchanges and their CHO, PRO,

FAT, and calorie values with a further breakdown of the items in each food group and their exchange values. It is easier to plan your diet when you understand the different food groups, their values, and how to fit them into your diet.

CONTENT OF FOOD EXCHANGES

Groups/Lists	Carbohydrate (g)	Protein (g)	Fat (g)	Calories
Carbohydrate Group				
Starch/Bread	15	3	0–1	80
Fruit	15	0	0	60
Milk				
Skim and very low fat	12	8	0–3	90
Low-fat	12	8	5	120
Whole	12	8	8	150
Other carbohydrates	15	varies	varies	varies
Vegetables	5	2	0	25
Meat and Meat Substitute Group				
Very lean	0	7	0–1	35
Lean	0	7	3	55
Medium-fat	0	7	5	75
High-fat	0	7	8	100
Fat Group	0	0	5	45

As you can see from the table, one starch/bread exchange contains 15 grams (about ½ ounce) of carbohydrate; a serving of fruit, 15 grams of carbohydrate; and a serving of vegetables, 5 grams of carbohydrate. This explains why your doctor or dietitian tells you to eat plenty of vegetables and less bread.

It is important to understand that when your dietitian says you can have two starch/bread exchanges at a meal, that means you have two choices from the starch/bread exchanges. You could have two slices of bread and use them for a sandwich, or you could have one slice of bread and another choice, such as a baked potato or one of the other carbohydrate items, or you might skip the bread and have the potato *and* the other carbohydrate item. The choice is up to you. This is why they are called exchanges, because you can exchange one food on the list for another one.

This is true also for the milk, fruit, and vegetable exchanges. If you are allowed two fruit exchanges, you may choose two different servings or double your serving unit, using, perhaps, 1 full cup of orange juice instead of ½ cup for breakfast. Most people use 2 or 3 ounces of the same kind of meat for a meal, although you can always use one or two ounces of meat and one ounce of cheese in a sandwich, or an ounce each of meat, cheese, fish, or poultry along with one egg in a big chef's salad.

The Exchange Lists are the basis of a meal planning system designed by a committee of the American Diabetes Association and the American Dietetic Association. While designed primarily for people with diabetes and others who must follow special diets, the Exchange Lists are based on principles of good nutrition that apply to everyone. © 1995 American Diabetes Association, Inc., The American Dietetic Association. Used with permission.

Throughout the following lists, items with 400 milligrams or more of sodium are identified by an asterisk (*).

Starch/Bread List Each item in this list, in the amount specified, contains 15 grams of carbohydrate, 3 grams of protein, 1 or less grams of fat, and 80 calories. Whenever possible, bread and cereal products should be whole-grain. Whole-grain products average about 2 grams of fiber per serving. Some foods are even higher in fiber.

You can choose your starch/bread exchanges from any of the items on this list. If you want to eat a starch/bread food that is not on this list, the general rule is that ½ cup of cereal, grain, or cooked pasta is one serving and 1 ounce of bread is one serving. Your dietitian can help you be more exact.

Cereals and grains

Bran cereals	½ cup
Bulgur	½ cup
Cereal, cooked	½ cup
Cereal, puffed	1½ cups
Cereal, ready-to-eat, unsweetened	¾ cup
Cornmeal, dry	3 tablespoons
Couscous	⅓ cup
Flour, dry	3 tablespoons
Granola, low-fat	¼ cup
Grape-Nuts	¼ cup
Grits	½ cup
Kasha	½ cup
Millet	¼ cup
Muesli	¼ cup
Oats	½ cup
Pasta	½ cup
Rice, brown or white, cooked	⅓ cup
Rice milk	½ cup
Wheat, shredded	½ cup
Wheat germ	3 tablespoons

Starchy vegetables

Baked beans	1/3 cup
Corn	1/2 cup
Corn on cob, medium	1 ear (5 ounces)
Mixed vegetables with corn, peas, or pasta	1 cup
Peas, green	1/2 cup
Plantain	1/2 cup
Potato, baked or boiled	1 small (3 ounces)
Potato, mashed	1/2 cup
Winter squash (acorn or butternut)	1 cup
Yams, sweet potatoes, plain	1/2 cup

Bread

Bagel	1/2 bagel (1 ounce)
Bread, reduced-calorie	2 slices (1 1/2 ounces)
Bread, white, whole-wheat, pumpernickel, rye	1 slice (1 ounce)
Bread sticks, crisp, 4" × 1/2"	2 (2/3 ounce)
English muffin	1/2
Hot dog or hamburger bun	1/2 (1 ounce)
Pita bread, 6" across	1/2
Raisin bread, unfrosted	1 slice (1 ounce)
Roll, plain	1 small (1 ounce)
Tortilla, corn, 6" across	1
Tortilla, flour, 7–8" across	1
Waffle, 4 1/2" square, reduced-fat	1

Crackers and snacks

Animal crackers	8
Graham crackers, 2 1/2" square	3
Matzoh	3/4 ounce
Melba toast	4 slices
Oyster crackers	24
Popcorn, popped, no fat added or low-fat microwaved	3 cups
Pretzels	3/4 ounce
Rice cakes, 4" across	2
Saltine-type crackers	6
Snack chips, fat-free (tortilla, potato)	15–20 (3/4 ounce)
Whole-wheat crackers with no added fat	2–5 (3/4 ounce)

Starchy foods prepared with fat

(Count as one starch/bread exchange plus one fat exchange.)

Biscuit, 2½" across	1
Chow mein noodles	½ cup
Corn bread, 2" cube	1 (2 ounces)
Cracker, round butter-type	6
Croutons	1 cup
French-fried potatoes	16–25 pieces (3 ounces)
Granola	¼ cup
Muffin, small	1 (1½ ounces)
Pancake, 4" across	2
Popcorn, microwave	3 cups
Sandwich crackers, cheese or peanut butter filling	3
Stuffing, bread, prepared	⅓ cup
Taco shell, 6" across	2
Waffle, 4½" square	1
Whole-wheat crackers, fat added	4–6 (1 ounce)

Dried beans, peas, and lentils

(Count as one starch/bread exchange plus one very lean meat exchange.)

Beans and peas (garbanzo, pinto, kidney, white, split, black-eyed)	½ cup
Lima beans	⅔ cup
Lentils	½ cup
Miso	3 tablespoons*

Meat List Each serving of meat or meat substitute on this list contains about 7 grams of protein. The amount of fat and number of calories vary, depending on what kind of meat or substitute you choose. The list is divided into four parts according to the amount of fat and calories: very lean, lean, medium-fat, and high-fat. The table below indicates values for 1 ounce (one meat exchange) of each type.

	Carbohydrate (g)	Protein (g)	Fat (g)	Calories
Very lean	0	7	0–1	35
Lean	0	7	3	55
Medium-fat	0	7	5	75
High-fat	0	7	8	100

Try to use more very lean, lean, and medium-fat meat, poultry, and fish in your meal plan. This will help decrease your fat intake and may help decrease your risk of heart disease. Foods in the high-fat group are high in saturated fat, cholesterol, and calories. You should limit your choices from the high-fat group to three times per week. Meat and meat substitutes do not contribute any fiber to your meal plan. Meats should be weighed after they are cooked and have the bones and fat removed.

Very lean meat and substitutes (0 grams of carbohydrate, 7 grams of protein, 0–1 grams of fat, and 35 calories)

(One very lean meat exchange is equal to any one of the following items.)

Poultry:	Chicken or turkey (white meat, no skin), Cornish hen (no skin)	1 ounce
Fish:	Fresh or frozen cod, flounder, haddock, halibut, trout; tuna fresh or canned in water	1 ounce
Shellfish:	Clams, crab, lobster, scallops, shrimp, imitation shellfish	1 ounce
Game:	Duck or pheasant (no skin), venison, buffalo, ostrich	1 ounce
Cheese with 1 gram or less fat per ounce:	Nonfat or low-fat cottage cheese	1/4 cup
	Fat-free cheese	1 ounce
Other:	Processed sandwich meats with 1 gram or less fat per ounce, such as deli thin, shaved meats*, chipped beef*, turkey, ham	1 ounce
	Egg whites	2
	Egg substitutes, plain	1/4 cup
	Hot dogs* with 1 gram or less fat per ounce	1 ounce
	Kidney (high in cholesterol)	1 ounce
	Sausage with 1 gram or less fat per ounce	1 ounce

(Count as one very lean meat and one starch exchange.)

	Dried beans, peas, lentils (cooked)	1/2 cup

Lean meat and substitutes (0 grams of carbohydrate, 7 grams of protein, 3 grams of fat, and 55 calories)

(One exchange is equal to any one of the following items.)

Beef:	USDA Select or Choice grades of lean beef trimmed of fat, such as round, sirloin, and flank steak; tenderloin; roast (rib, chuck, rump); steak (T-bone, porterhouse, cubed), ground round	1 ounce
Lamb:	Roast, chop, leg	1 ounce
Pork:	Lean pork such as fresh ham; canned, cured, or boiled ham, Canadian bacon*, tenderloin, center loin chop	1 ounce
Veal:	Lean chops and roasts	1 ounce
Poultry:	Chicken, turkey (dark meat, no skin), chicken white meat (with skin), domestic duck or goose (well-drained of fat, no skin)	1 ounce
Fish:	Herring (uncreamed or smoked)	1 ounce
	Oysters	6 medium
	Salmon (fresh or canned), catfish	1 ounce
	Sardines (canned)	2 medium
	Tuna (canned in oil, drained)	¼ cup
Game:	Goose (no skin), rabbit	1 ounce
Cheese:	4.5%-fat cottage cheese	¼ cup
	Grated Parmesan	2 tablespoons
	Cheeses with 3 grams or less fat per ounce	1 ounce
Other:	Hot dogs with 3 grams or less fat per ounce*	1½ ounces
	Processed sandwich meat with 3 grams or less fat per ounce, such as turkey pastrami or kielbasa	1 ounce
	Liver, heart (high in cholesterol)	1 ounce

Medium-fat meat and substitutes (0 grams of carbohydrate, 7 grams of protein, 5 grams of fat, and 75 calories)

(One exchange is equal to any one of the following items.)

Beef:	Most beef products fall into this category (ground beef, meat loaf, corned beef, short ribs, Prime grades of meat trimmed of fat, such as prime rib)	1 ounce
Pork:	Top loin, chop, Boston butt, cutlets	1 ounce

Lamb:	Rib roast, ground	1 ounce
Veal:	Cutlet (ground or cubed, unbreaded)	1 ounce
Poultry:	Chicken dark meat (with skin), ground turkey or ground chicken, fried chicken (with skin)	1 ounce
Fish:	Any fried fish product	1 ounce
Cheese:	With 5 grams or less fat per ounce:	
	Feta	1 ounce
	Mozzarella	1 ounce
	Ricotta	1/4 cup (2 ounces)
Other:	Egg (high in cholesterol, limit to 3 per week)	1
	Sausage with 5 grams or less fat per ounce	1 ounce
	Soy milk	1 cup
	Tempeh	1/4 cup
	Tofu	4 ounces or 1/2 cup

High-fat meat and substitutes (0 grams of carbohydrate, 7 grams of protein, 8 grams of fat, and 100 calories)

Remember, these items are high in saturated fat, cholesterol, and calories and may raise blood cholesterol if eaten on a regular basis. (One high-fat exchange is equal to any one of the following items.)

Pork:	Spareribs, ground pork, pork sausage	1 ounce
Cheese:	All regular cheese,* such as American, cheddar, Monterey Jack, Swiss	1 ounce
Other:	Processed sandwich meats with 8 grams or more fat per ounce, such as bologna, pimento loaf, salami	1 ounce
	Sausage, such as bratwurst, Italian, knockwurst, Polish, smoked	1 ounce
	Hot dog (turkey or chicken)*	1 (10 to the pound)
	Bacon	3 slices (20 slices to the pound)

(Count as one high-fat meat plus one fat exchange.)

| | Hot dog (beef, pork, or combination)* | 1 (10 to the pound) |
| | Peanut butter (contains unsaturated fat) | 2 tablespoons |

Vegetable List One serving of each vegetable listed below contains 5 grams of carbohydrate, 2 grams of protein, 0 grams of fat, 25 calories, and 2–3 grams of dietary fiber.

Vegetables are a good source of vitamins and minerals. Fresh and frozen vegetables have more vitamins and less added salt than canned vegetables; rinsing canned vegetables will remove much of the salt.

Unless otherwise noted, the serving size for vegetables (one vegetable exchange) is ½ cup cooked vegetables or vegetable juice, or 1 cup of raw vegetables. If you eat one to two vegetable choices at a meal or snack, you do not have to count the calories or carbohydrates because they contain small amounts of these nutrients.

Artichoke
Artichoke hearts
Asparagus
Beans (green, wax, or
    Italian)
Bean sprouts
Beets
Broccoli
Brussels sprouts
Cabbage
Carrots
Cauliflower
Celery
Cucumber
Eggplant
Green onions or
    scallions
Greens (collard, kale,
    mustard, turnip)
Kohlrabi
Leeks

Mixed vegetables (without corn,
    peas, or pasta)
Mushrooms
Okra
Onions
Pea pods
Peppers, all varieties
Radishes
Salad greens (endive, escarole,
    lettuce, romaine, spinach)
Sauerkraut*
Spinach
Summer squash
Tomato
Tomatoes, canned
Tomato sauce*
Tomato/vegetable juice*
Turnips
Water chestnuts
Watercress
Zucchini

Starchy vegetables such as beans, corn, peas, and potatoes are included in the starch/bread list.

Fruit List Each item on this list, in the amount specified, contains about 15 grams of carbohydrate and 60 calories. Fresh, frozen, and dried fruits have about 2 grams of fiber per serving. The carbohydrate and calorie contents are based on a typical serving of the most commonly eaten fruits. You should use fresh fruit or fruit frozen without added sugar. Whole fruit is more filling than fruit juice and may be a better choice for those who are trying to lose weight. The weight includes skin, core, seeds, and rind.

Fruit

Apple, unpeeled, small	1 (4 ounces)
Applesauce, unsweetened	1/2 cup
Apples, dried	4 rings
Apricots, fresh	4 whole (5 1/2 ounces)
Apricots, canned	1/2 cup
Apricots, dried	8 halves
Banana, small	1 (4 ounces)
Blackberries	1/4 cup
Blueberries	1/4 cup
Cantaloupe, small	1/3 melon (11 ounces) or 1 cup cubes
Cherries, sweet, fresh	12 (3 ounces)
Cherries, sweet, canned	1/2 cup
Dates	3
Figs, fresh	1 1/2 large or 2 medium (3 1/2 ounces)
Figs, dried	1 1/2 cups
Fruit cocktail	1/2 cup
Grapefruit, large	1/2 (11 ounces)
Grapefruit sections, canned	3/4 cup
Grapes, small	17 (3 ounces)
Honeydew melon	1 slice (10 ounces) or 1 cup cubes
Kiwi	1 (3 1/2 ounces)
Mandarin oranges, canned	3/4 cup
Mango, small	1/2 fruit (5 1/2 ounces) or 1/2 cup
Nectarine, small	1 (5 ounces)
Orange, small	1 (6 1/2 ounces)
Papaya	1/2 fruit (8 ounces) or 1 cup cubes
Peach, medium, fresh	1 (6 ounces)
Peaches, canned	1/2 cup
Pear, large, fresh	1/2 (4 ounces)
Pears, canned	1/2 cup
Pineapple, fresh	3/4 cup
Pineapple, canned	1/2 cup
Plum, small	2 (5 ounces)
Plums, canned	1/2 cup
Prunes, dried	3
Raisins	2 tablespoons
Raspberries	1 cup
Strawberries	1 1/4 cups whole berries
Tangerine, small	2 (8 ounces)
Watermelon	1 slice (13 1/2 ounces) or 1 1/4 cups cubes

Fruit juice

Apple juice or cider	1/2 cup
Cranberry juice cocktail	1/3 cup
Cranberry juice cocktail, reduced-calorie	1 cup
Fruit juice blends, 100% juice	1/3 cup
Grape juice	1/3 cup
Grapefruit juice	1/2 cup
Orange juice	1/2 cup
Pineapple juice	1/2 cup
Prune juice	1/3 cup

Milk List Each serving of milk or milk products on this list contains 12 grams of carbohydrate and 8 grams of protein. The amount of fat in milk is measured in percent of butterfat. That amount, like the number of calories, depends on the kind of milk. The list is divided into three parts, according to the amount of fat and calories: skim and very low fat milk, low-fat milk, and whole milk. The following table shows values for one serving (one milk exchange) of each category.

	Carbohydrate (g)	Protein (g)	Fat (g)	Calories
Skim and very low fat	12	8	0–3	90
Low-fat	12	8	5	120
Whole	12	8	8	150

Milk is a very important source of protein and calcium, the mineral needed for growth and repair of bones. Yogurt is also a good source of protein and calcium. Yogurt and many dry or powdered milk products have different amounts of fat. If you have questions about the fat and calorie content of a particular item, read the nutrition information.

Milk is good not only alone as a beverage, but also added to cereal and other foods. The higher the fat content of milk and yogurt, the greater the amount of saturated fat and cholesterol. Choose lower-fat varieties. One cup of milk equals 8 fluid ounces or 1/2 pint.

Skim and very low fat milk

Skim milk	1 cup
1/2% milk	1 cup
1% milk	1 cup
Nonfat or low-fat buttermilk	1 cup
Evaporated skim milk	1/2 cup

Nonfat dry milk	1/3 cup dry
Plain nonfat yogurt	3/4 cup
Nonfat or low-fat, fruit-flavored yogurt sweetened with aspartame or with a nonnutritive sweetener	1 cup

Low-fat milk

2% milk	1 cup
Plain low-fat yogurt	3/4 cup
Sweet acidophilus milk	1 cup

Whole milk

Whole milk	1 cup
Evaporated whole milk	1/2 cup
Goat's milk	1 cup
Kefir	1 cup

Fat List One serving (the amount specified) of each item on the fat list has 5 grams of fat and 45 calories. In general one fat exchange is 1 teaspoon of regular margarine or vegetable oil, or 1 tablespoon of regular salad dressing.

All fats are high in calories and should be carefully measured. Everyone should modify fat intake by eating unsaturated fats instead of saturated fats. The sodium content of the foods listed here varies widely; check product labels for precise information.

Monounsaturated fats

Avocado, medium	1/8 avocado (1 ounce)
Nuts	
Almonds and cashews	6 nuts
Mixed nuts (50% peanuts)	6 nuts
Peanuts	10 nuts
Pecans	4 halves
Oil (canola, olive, peanut)	1 teaspoon
Olives: ripe (black)	8 large
green, stuffed*	10 large
Peanut butter, smooth or crunchy	2 teaspoons
Sesame seeds	1 tablespoon
Tahini paste	2 teaspoons

Polyunsaturated fats

| Margarine: stick, tub, or squeeze | 1 teaspoon |
| lower-fat (30% to 50% vegetable oil) | 1 tablespoon |

Mayonnaise: regular	1 teaspoon
reduced-fat	1 tablespoon
Nuts, walnuts, English	4 halves
Oil (corn, safflower, soybean)	1 teaspoon
Salad dressing: regular*	1 tablespoon
reduced-fat	2 tablespoons
Miracle Whip Salad Dressing: regular	2 teaspoons
reduced-fat	1 tablespoon
Seeds: pumpkin, sunflower	1 tablespoon

Saturated fats

Bacon, cooked	1 slice (20 slices to the pound)
Bacon, grease	1 teaspoon
Butter, stick	1 teaspoon
Butter, whipped	2 teaspoons
Butter, reduced-fat	1 tablespoon
Chitterlings, boiled	2 tablespoons ($^1/_2$ ounce)
Coconut, sweetened, shredded	2 tablespoons
Cream, half and half	2 tablespoons
Cream cheese, regular	1 tablespoon ($^1/_2$ ounce)
Cream cheese, reduced-fat	2 tablespoons (1 ounce)
Shortening or lard	1 teaspoon
Sour cream, regular	2 tablespoons
Sour cream, reduced-fat	3 tablespoons
Fatback or salt pork* (see below)†	$^1/_4$ ounce

† Use a piece 1" × 1" × $^1/_4$" if you plan to eat the fatback cooked with vegetables. Use a piece 2" × 1" × $^1/_2$" when eating only the vegetables with the fatback removed.

Free Foods A free food is any food or drink that contains fewer than 20 calories per serving. You may eat as much as you want of the items listed here that have no serving size specified, and 2 or 3 servings per day of items that have a specified serving size. Be sure to spread them out through the day. See vegetable list for free vegetables.

Drinks

Bouillon*, broth consommé*	Coffee or tea (without sugar)
Low-sodium bouillon or broth	Club soda
Carbonated or mineral water	Diet soft drinks, sugar-free
Unsweetened cocoa powder	Sugar-free drink mixes
(1 tablespoon)	Sugar-free tonic water

Sugar-free or low-sugar foods

Sugar-free hard candy (1 candy)
Sugar-free gelatin
Unflavored gelatin
Sugar-free gum

Jams and jellies, low sugar or light (2 teaspoons)
Sugar-free pancake syrup (2 tablespoons)

Sugar substitutes, alternatives, or replacements that are approved by the Food and Drug Administration (FDA) are safe to use. Common brand names include:

Equal (aspartame)
Sprinkle Sweet (saccharin)
Sweet One (acesulfame K)

Sweet-10 (saccharin)
Sugar Twin (saccharin)
Sweet 'n Low (saccharin)

Condiments

Catsup (1 tablespoon)
Dill pickles*
Horseradish
Lemon juice
Lime juice

Mustard
Soy sauce*, regular or light
Taco sauce (1 tablespoon)
Vinegar

Fat-free or reduced-fat foods

Cream cheese, fat-free	1 tablespoon
Creamers, nondairy, liquid	1 tablespoon
Creamers, nondairy, powdered	2 teaspoons
Mayonnaise, fat-free	1 tablespoon
Mayonnaise, reduced-fat	1 teaspoon
Margarine, fat-free	4 tablespoons
Margarine, reduced-fat	1 teaspoon
Miracle Whip, nonfat	1 tablespoon
Miracle Whip, reduced-fat	1 teaspoon
Nonstick cooking spray	
Salad dressing, fat-free	1 tablespoon
Salad dressing, fat-free, Italian	2 tablespoons
Salsa	1/4 cup
Sour cream, fat-free, reduced-fat	1 tablespoon
Whipped topping, regular or light	2 tablespoons

Seasonings

Seasonings can help make food taste better, but you must be careful of sodium levels. Be careful with seasonings that contain sodium or are salts, such as garlic or celery salt, and lemon pepper.

Flavoring extracts	Spices
Garlic	Tabasco or hot pepper sauce
Herbs, fresh or dried	Wine, used in cooking
Pimento	Worcestershire sauce

Other Carbohydrates One exchange equals 15 grams carbohydrate, or starch, or one fruit, or one milk serving. Moderate amounts of some foods can be used in your meal plan in spite of their sugar or fat content, as long as you maintain blood sugar control. The following list gives average exchange values for some of these foods. Notice that because they are concentrated sources of carbohydrate, serving sizes are very small. Check with your dietitian for advice on how often you can eat such foods and read the nutrition facts on food labels.

Food	*Exchanges*
$^1/_{12}$ angel food cake, unfrosted	2 carbohydrates
2" square brownie, unfrosted	1 carbohydrate and 1 fat
2" square cake, unfrosted	1 carbohydrate and 1 fat
2" square cake, frosted	2 carbohydrates and 1 fat
2 small cookies, fat-free	1 carbohydrate
2 small cookies or 1 sandwich cookie with creme filling	1 carbohydrate and 1 fat
5 vanilla wafers	1 carbohydrate and 1 fat
1 small cupcake, frosted	2 carbohydrates and 1 fat
$^1/_4$ cup cranberry sauce, jellied	$1^1/_2$ carbohydrates
1 medium ($1^1/_2$ ounces) doughnut, plain cake	$1^1/_2$ carbohydrates and 2 fats
$3^3/_4$" across (2 ounces) doughnut, glazed	2 carbohydrates and 2 fats
1 bar (3 ounces) fruit juice bar, frozen, 100% juice	1 carbohydrate
1 roll ($^3/_4$ ounce) fruit snack, chewy (pureed fruit concentrate)	1 carbohydrate
1 tablespoon fruit spread, 100% fruit	1 carbohydrate
$^1/_2$ cup gelatin, regular	1 carbohydrate
3 gingersnaps	1 carbohydrate
1 granola bar	1 carbohydrate and 1 fat
1 granola bar, fat-free	2 carbohydrates
$^1/_3$ cup hummus	1 carbohydrate and 1 fat
$^1/_2$ cup ice cream	1 carbohydrate and 2 fats
$^1/_2$ cup ice cream, light	1 carbohydrate and 1 fat
$^1/_2$ cup ice cream, fat-free, no sugar added	1 carbohydrate
1 tablespoon jam or jelly, regular	1 carbohydrate
1 cup, milk, chocolate, whole	2 carbohydrates and 1 fat
$^1/_6$ pie, fruit, 2 crusts	3 carbohydrates and 2 fats

1/8 pie, pumpkin or custard	1 carbohydrate and 2 fats
12–18 (1 ounce) potato chips	1 carbohydrate and 2 fats
1/2 cup pudding, regular, made with low-fat milk	2 carbohydrates
1/2 cup pudding, sugar-free, made with low-fat milk	1 carbohydrate
1/4 cup salad dressing, fat-free*	1 carbohydrate
1/2 cup sherbet, sorbet	2 carbohydrates
1/2 cup spaghetti or pasta sauce, canned*	1 carbohydrate and 1 fat
1 (2 1/2 ounces) sweet roll or danish	2 1/2 carbohydrates and 2 fats
2 tablespoons syrup, light	1 carbohydrate
1 tablespoon syrup, regular	1 carbohydrate
1/4 cup syrup, regular	4 carbohydrates
6–12 (1 ounce) tortilla chips	1 carbohydrate and 2 fats
1/3 cup yogurt, frozen, low-fat, fat-free	1 carbohydrate and 0–1 fat
1/2 cup yogurt, frozen, fat-free, no sugar added	1 carbohydrate
1 cup yogurt, low-fat with fruit	3 carbohydrates and 0–1 fat

Some food you buy uncooked will weigh less after you cook it. Starches often swell in cooking, so a small amount of uncooked starch will become a much larger amount of cooked food. The following table shows some of the changes.

Food (Starch Group)	Uncooked	Cooked
Oatmeal	3 tablespoons	1/2 cup
Cream of Wheat	2 tablespoons	1/2 cup
Grits	3 tablespoons	1/2 cup
Rice	2 tablespoons	1/3 cup
Spaghetti	1/4 cup	1/2 cup
Noodles	1/3 cup	1/2 cup
Macaroni	1/4 cup	1/2 cup
Dried beans	1/4 cup	1/2 cup
Dried peas	1/4 cup	1/2 cup
Lentils	3 tablespoons	1/2 cup

CHAPTER 4

Ingredients

WE WANT COOKING to be a fun and simple experience for you and your family. That is why we recommend, as much as possible, that you prepare foods the same for all members of your family. Everyone can benefit from the healthy nutrition principles of a meal plan for diabetes, which includes eating moderate amounts of protein, fats, and carbohydrates. There may be times, however, when the person with diabetes prefers special, lower-sugar foods. It is a good idea to keep the foods you use frequently on hand.

We have tried to only use ingredients that are nationally available, and many that you may be using already. New products appear in the supermarket almost daily. As with any food, you will have to experiment to find your favorites. Many foods on the market are labeled diet or diabetic or sugar-free. Be sure to check the labels carefully on these foods and compare the calorie and carbohydrate amount to the original food. It is not uncommon to find "diet" food with just as many grams of carbohydrate as the original product at a not so "diet" price.

Many foods in the grocery store have labels that can sometimes be confusing. To help you navigate the grocery aisles, we have included a list of common terms and label definitions as established by the Food and Drug Administration.

TERMS COMMONLY USED ON LABELS

Sugar

Sugar-Free: Less than 0.5 gram of sugar per serving.

No Added Sugar, Without Added Sugar, No Sugar Added: These are not the same as "sugar-free." A label with this wording indicates that no sugars were added during processing, or that processing does not increase the sugar content above the amount the ingredient naturally contains. Check the nutrition label to see the total amount of sugar in the product.

Reduced Sugar: At least 25% less sugar per serving than the regular product.

Calories

Calorie-Free: Fewer than 5 calories per serving.

Low-Calorie: 40 calories or less per serving. (If servings are smaller than 30 grams, or smaller than 2 tablespoons, this means 40 calories or less per 50 grams of food.)

Reduced-Calorie, Fewer Calories: At least 25% fewer calories per serving than the regular product.

Fat

Fat-Free, Nonfat: Less than 0.5 gram of fat per serving.

Low-fat: 3 grams or less of fat per serving. (If servings are smaller than 30 grams, or smaller than 2 tablespoons, this means 3 grams or less of fat per 50 grams of food.)

Reduced-Fat, Less Fat: At least 25% less fat per serving than the regular product.

Cholesterol

Cholesterol-Free: Less than 2 milligrams of cholesterol, and 2 grams or less of saturated fat per serving.

Low-Cholesterol: 20 milligrams or less of cholesterol, and 2 grams or less of saturated fat per serving.

Reduced-Cholesterol, Less Cholesterol: At least 25% less cholesterol, and 2 grams or less of saturated fat per serving than the regular product.

Sodium

Sodium-Free: Less than 5 milligrams of sodium per serving.

Low-Sodium: 140 milligrams or less of sodium per serving.

Very Low Sodium: 35 milligrams or less of sodium per serving.

Reduced-Sodium, Less Sodium: At least 25% less sodium per serving than the regular product.

Light or Lite Foods

Foods that are labeled "Light" or "Lite" are usually lower in fat or lower in calories than the regular product. In order to make the claim, a food must have 33.3% fewer calories or 50% less fat per serving than the original food. Check the nutrition label on the product to make sure.

INGREDIENTS USED FREQUENTLY

Low-Calorie Sweeteners

There are numerous low-calorie sweeteners or sugar substitutes available on the market today. Some work better in certain cooking than others. For example, Splenda and Sweet One tend to be more heat stable for baking, while Equal is good in gelatins and cold dishes. It really is a matter of personal preference. One teaspoon of sugar contains four grams of carbohydrates and 15 calories while one teaspoon of a low-calorie sweetener contains almost no calories or carbohydrate grams. You need to decide what works best for you. You will find that some of the recipes in this book use sugar substitutes while others do not. We have tried to make most of the desserts in this book yield 15 grams of carbohydrate per serving. Therefore, we used different combinations of sugar, natural sweeteners, and sugar substitutes to give us the best results, both nutritionally and taste-wise.

There are currently four low-calorie sweeteners approved for use in the United States. These are: acesulfame K, aspartame (Equal and NutraSweet), saccharin (Sugar Twin and Sweet 'n Low), and sucralose (Splenda). They are considered low-calorie sweeteners because they give food or beverages a sweet taste without adding calories or carbohydrates. For those of you wanting to use a sugar substitute, the following information will help you determine how much to add in your recipes.

We're sure you will agree that we should fit the sugar substitutes, including the liquid ones that some people prefer, to our own preferences. The following table will help you decide how much sugar substitute you need for your recipes.

Sugar Substitutes and Equivalents

1 teaspoon sugar =	1 teaspoon Sugar Twin
	1 Equal tablet
	1/2 packet Equal or NutraSweet
	1/10 teaspoon Sweet 'n Low
	1 teaspoon Equal Spoonful
	1 teaspoon Splenda

1 tablespoon sugar =	1 tablespoon Sugar Twin
	1½ packets Equal or NutraSweet
	⅓ teaspoon Sweet 'n Low
	1 tablespoon Equal Spoonful
	1 tablespoon Splenda
¼ cup sugar =	¼ cup Sugar Twin
	6 packets Equal or NutraSweet
	1½ teaspoons Sweet 'n Low
	¼ cup Equal Spoonful
	¼ cup Splenda
½ cup sugar =	½ cup Sugar Twin
	12 packets Equal or NutraSweet
	1 tablespoon Sweet 'n Low
	½ cup Equal Spoonful
	½ cup Splenda
¾ cup sugar =	¼ cup Sugar Twin
	18 packets Equal or NutraSweet
	1½ tablespoons Sweet 'n Low
	¾ cup Equal Spoonful
	¾ cup Splenda
1 cup sugar =	1 cup Sugar Twin
	24 packets Equal or NutraSweet
	2 tablespoons Sweet 'n Low
	1 cup Equal Spoonful
	1 cup Splenda

Sugar

It is much easier to prepare good cakes or cookies now that we can have some sugar in our diets. Like fat, sugar improves the texture of these baked goods. Cakes made without sugar have the texture of coarse muffins. There are several forms of sugar: sucrose, which we know as table sugar; lactose, which is found in milk; and fructose, which is found in fruit and honey. All of them will raise your blood sugar (glucose) level. We know that we can have a small amount of sugar in our diets, with our doctor's permission. That doesn't mean we can now load our cereal or coffee with sugar, but it does mean we can enjoy a few more desserts.

As you are preparing food, remember that it is the total carbohydrate that matters most in your meals, instead of the source of the carbohydrate. The days are gone when people with diabetes had to avoid sugar completely. When cooking and baking, it is important to keep in mind the role of sugar. Sugar provides sweetness, structure, texture, color, moistness, tenderness, and shelf stability to food. This means when used in baking, it makes cakes moist, frosting sweet, breads golden brown with a crispy crust, and helps jams and jellies keep from spoiling.

Besides granulated white sugar, other common forms and sources of sugar include: brown sugar, corn syrup, molasses, powdered sugar, fruits, fruit purees and fruit juices.

Many traditional dessert recipes are so high in sugar that you can often take some out without altering the flavor very much. In fact, many people find they enjoy the newer, lighter flavor better.

Besides using low-calorie sweeteners in your recipes, the following are a few ways to reduce the sugar in your baking:

- Omit all of the sugar if a recipe has enough fruit in it to stand on its own. This may be the case if you are preparing a fruit crisp or cobbler. The riper the fruit, the more sweet taste it will provide.
- Reduce the amount of sugar you include in a recipe. Many times you can reduce sugar by one-fourth in a recipe without any noticeable changes. If you find this reduction provides a satisfactory dessert, try reducing the amount of sugar by one-third or up to one-half the next time you prepare the item. We recommend doing this gradually. You may want to try using superfine sugar to help keep the dessert light and tender. Some professional bakers also prefer using cane versus beet sugar for its baking properties.
- Use flavorings that bring out the natural sweetness in foods. Spices and flavorings like cinnamon, nutmeg, cloves, and vanilla and almond extract can enhance the sweetness in foods without the need for added sugar.
- Sprinkle small amounts of white or brown sugar, drizzle honey, or shave chocolate onto the top of a dessert in which you have reduced the sugar content. Since this is the first part of the dessert that you typically taste, you will get the sensation of sweetness without the added calories and carbohydrates.

Nonfat Instant Dry Milk and Dry Buttermilk

Dry milk is easy to store, is fat-free, and dissolves easily in liquid, blends well into baked products, doesn't have to be scalded to make bread, and doesn't have to be refrigerated until it is mixed with liquid. You can buy dry milk by the twenty-quart package; pour the powder into an empty gallon jar and keep it in your kitchen, along with flour and sugar, where it is handy whenever you need it. Dry milk has all of the nutrients of fat-free milk without the bulk.

Dry buttermilk has all of the advantages of instant dry milk except that you have to keep the powder refrigerated after it is opened.

If you don't want to use dry milk when it's called for in a recipe, you may generally substitute fresh milk for the liquid in the recipe. When using fresh milk always purchase fat-free milk, because that is what the nutritive values are based on.

Give instant dry milk or dry buttermilk a try if you've never used them before. We think you will find them as easy to use as fresh milk, and generally less expensive.

Eggs and Egg Substitutes

Eggs or egg substitutes are necessary in most cakes and cookies, and we have used them in these recipes because they don't contain any carbohydrate and they improve the texture of the cakes and cookies. We have included notes after each recipe telling you how to adapt the recipes for low-cholesterol and/or low-sodium diets since many people with diabetes are following those diets. If they cannot be adapted for low-cholesterol or low-sodium diets, we note that also. Most dessert recipes can use egg whites or liquid egg substitute instead of eggs, but occasionally they don't give good results and in those cases we haven't put them in the statement of substitutes for the ingredients.

We generally use Egg Beaters as a liquid egg substitute but there are several other good brands.

Low-Sodium Foods and Salt

Some recipes are too high in sodium for some people's diets, but you can't delete any of the ingredients without ruining the dish, so in these cases we have just stated that it may not be suitable for those on a low-sodium diet. Low-sodium baking powder can be substituted for regular baking powder, but there isn't any suitable substitute for baking soda. Salt-free margarine is available and there isn't any sodium in vegetable oil, which is used in many recipes.

Salt is typically used in baking to add a salty taste, enhance other flavors, and allow the food to have a longer shelf life. A little salt typically goes a long way in recipes. In fact, studies have shown that salt has more impact on foods when it's baked or cooked into a product than when it is added on top.

In most dessert recipes you can omit the salt without causing a change in the recipe taste or texture. As you use less salt in your diet, you may find that the natural flavors of foods are more noticeable and enjoyable. If the recipe seems to lack flavor after you have reduced or eliminated the salt, try increasing the amount of spices in the recipe to enhance other flavors.

Fats

Margarine and vegetable oil are used in most of the recipes in this book. Occasionally, we have used butter in recipes where it has dramatically enhanced the flavor of the dessert without contributing too many fat calories. As with all cooking ingredients, fat plays an important role in the making of a successful recipe.

Fat provides flavor, moistness, tenderness, body and fluffiness, a rich creamy texture, an even blending of flavors, heat stability, and an enhanced taste to foods. Different types of fat have different cooking properties. This means that cookies made with oil may turn out very different from cookies made with butter or margarine, even though they both contain the same total amount of fat.

We get fat in our diet and in our baking from a number of sources. These can include butter, margarine, oils, coconut, peanut butter, nuts and seeds, shortenings, lard, and mayonnaise. There are also fats in whole milk products like creams, cream cheese, other cheeses, and ice cream, and in bacon, other meats, and avocados.

People need a certain amount of fat in their diet. Fat provides key nutrients for the body and helps you feel satisfied after eating. Fat used in moderation is part of healthy eating.

Many times, however, traditional recipes are very high in fat. Reducing the fat in baked products can be a bit tricky because the fat is needed to add lightness and texture to cookies, breads, cakes, and pastries. A cookie made with too little fat will be hard and a cake made without adequate fat will resemble a poor muffin. Therefore, some people may opt to reduce fat in other parts of their diets rather than take it out of their favorite desserts. Others find they can reduce the fat in most recipes by one-fourth without much noticeable difference. Our best advice is to experiment and adjust recipes to your personal tastes and preferences.

If you reduce the fat in a recipe and find that the batter seems too heavy, you can sometimes compensate by using a little less flour, or by using cake flour instead of all-purpose flour. Take care not to overmix the batter, as this just makes it heavier. This is especially true when making bars and muffins.

Sometimes you can use a fruit puree or applesauce to replace some of the fat in a recipe. The fruit yields a very moist product. However, because the food tends to be heavier in consistency, you may need to slightly increase baking time.

When adjusting the fat in a recipe, we recommend that you do it a little at a time. Make notes next to your recipe about the changes you made and how the final dessert turned out. Then, the next time you prepare that food item, you can decide if you want to make further changes.

When baking with fats and oils, it is best if they are at room temperature. Margarine and butter will work best if taken out of the refrigerator about 30 minutes before using. Vegetable oil should be kept in a cool, dry place, at about 70°F, until it is used. You do not need to refrigerate oil unless you expect to keep it several months; bring it back to room temperature before using it.

Oat Bran
Oat bran may be helpful in normalizing blood sugar. It is included in several recipes in this book. We are advocates of increasing fiber in the diet and oat bran is one way to do this. Wheat bran is also an excellent source of fiber and can be added to recipes to boost fiber.

Flours
It is important to use the type of flour called for in each recipe. Bread flour is higher in gluten than all-purpose flour and reacts differently in baking. It holds more water than all-purpose flour, so a recipe using bread flour may not work well when you use some other kind of flour. Most of the recipes included in this book use all-purpose flour, but there are times when bread or cake flour is indicated to yield better results. You can keep flour refrigerated or frozen if you are not going to use it soon. Just remember to bring it back to room temperature before using it in baking.

CHAPTER 5

Cakes

WE FEEL BAD when we think of all the people with diabetes who went without a birthday cake over the years because we didn't know how to work these special foods successfully into the meal plan. Now, with the use of carbohydrate counting and closer glucose monitoring, anyone can easily make cake, and even ice cream, a part of their lives.

With the increasing knowledge of how carbohydrates affect blood sugar, we are able to use a larger variety of ingredients in cooking and baking. In addition, tastier sugar-type substitutes are available for those wishing to use them.

However, a cake is still a cake, and there are some basic guidelines for preparing them in order to achieve good quality. This is especially true if you are using fruits or fruit purees in place of some of the original fat or sugar in the recipe. The following guidelines are particularly important when you are making cakes:

1. A cake is a delicately balanced formula and following the directions carefully will help yield a good product. When you are preparing a cake for someone with diabetes, it is best to avoid adding extra items to the recipe unless you recalculate the grams of carbohydrate, carbohydrate choices, or food exchanges for the final product. To avoid adding extra carbohydrates and sugar, these cakes are generally not frosted. If you choose to add frosting, remember to count additional grams of carbohydrate, carbohydrate choices, or food exchanges. Sometimes a dollop of lite or fat-free whipped topping or a fruit sauce

such as unsweetened applesauce on a spice cake is a tasty substitute for frosting.

2. Standard measuring cups and spoons should be used and the cakes should be baked at the temperature specified in the recipe.

3. Do not sift flour unless sifted flour is specified in the recipe, since the weight of sifted versus unsifted flour is different. Also, always use the type of flour called for; cake, all-purpose, and bread flours have different compositions and produce different results.

4. Ingredients should be at room temperature unless the recipe specifies chilled. This is particularly true of margarine, eggs, and liquid egg substitutes. I keep reserved flour, nuts, dates, raisins, and other items in the freezer, but I always bring them to room temperature before using them.

5. If you want to bake your cake in a different-sized pan from that specified in the recipe, fill the new pan two-thirds full, and you may need to change the baking time also. If there is not enough batter in a pan, the resulting cake will be thin and hard; if there is too much batter, it may spill over the sides of the pan and create a mess in the oven.

6. If you are making a single cake, put the cake pan in the center of the oven. If you are making a layer cake, place the pans on the same shelf if possible. Be careful that they do not touch each other, so the heat will circulate freely and uniformly around them.

7. Avoid changing the portion size of the cake without taking into account the effect on food exchanges, If, for example, you double a serving size, you are also doubling the number of carbohydrate grams or choices or food exchanges. The exchanges listed are based only on the portion size indicated in the recipe.

8. All baking times assume preheated ovens.

9. Nonstick cake pans make it easy to turn your cake out of the pan after it is baked. This is particularly true for loaf cakes, which are never cut in the pan the way some cakes are. I also prefer to prepare pans with a spray instead of greasing them. It is simpler and saves a few calories per serving.

Applesauce Cake

This cake is a favorite of our neighbor Johnathan Franks. As he told me once, he is a bottomless pit when it comes to cake, cookies, and ice cream. When he first moved in next door, I used to give him candy but then I thought, "This is crazy, no dietitian should be giving neighbor children all that candy." So I talked to his mother, Jan, and we decided to stick to healthier cakes, cookies, low-fat milk, and foods with less fat and sugar in them . . . and he is just as happy with them as he was with the candy. This recipe is a good source of fiber.

1 cup 100% Bran, Fiber One, Bran Buds, or All-Bran	1 cup unsweetened applesauce
1 large egg	2 tablespoons water
¼ cup vegetable oil	1 cup all-purpose flour
Liquid sugar substitute equal to ½ cup sugar or the equivalent to ½ cup dry sugar substitute and 2 tablespoons water	1 teaspoon baking soda
	2 tablespoons dry buttermilk
	½ teaspoon salt
	1 teaspoon cinnamon
2 tablespoons packed brown sugar	¼ cup chopped pecans
	¼ cup raisins, washed and drained

Place bran, egg, vegetable oil, sugar substitute, brown sugar, apple-sauce, and water in mixer bowl. Mix lightly and let stand for 30 to 45 minutes. (This standing is very important to allow the cereal to soften.) Stir flour, soda, dry buttermilk, salt, and cinnamon together to blend. Add flour mixture to bran mixture and mix at medium speed to blend well. Add pecans and raisins. Spread the batter evenly in a well-greased 9 × 5-inch loaf pan.

Bake at 375°F for about 45 minutes, or until a cake tester comes out clean from the center and the cake pulls away from the sides of the pan. Cool in the pan for 10 minutes and then turn out onto a wire rack and cool to room temperature. Cut into 14 equal slices and use 1 slice per serving.

Yield: 14 (1-slice) servings
Food exchanges per serving: 1 starch and 1 fat; or 1 carbohydrate choice
Sugar per serving: 2 teaspoons or 9 grams
Low-cholesterol diets: Omit egg. Use ¼ cup liquid egg substitute.
Low-sodium diets: Omit salt.
Nutritive values per serving:

Calories: 124	FAT: 6 g
CHO: 15 g	Na: 197 mg
PRO: 3 g	Cholesterol: 15 mg

Chocolate Cake

This cake can also be baked in a 9 × 13-inch cake pan. The cake will be thinner but the good flavor will remain, and if you cut it into 16 equal pieces, the nutritive values will remain the same.

1¼ cups all-purpose flour	½ teaspoon cinnamon
⅓ cup unsweetened cocoa powder	½ teaspoon salt
⅓ cup sugar	2 teaspoons baking powder
Dry sugar substitute equal to ½ cup sugar	1 cup water at room temperature
	2 large eggs
2 tablespoons instant nonfat dry milk	⅓ cup vegetable oil
	1½ teaspoons vanilla extract

Place flour, cocoa, sugar, dry sugar substitute, dry milk, cinnamon, salt, and baking powder in a mixer bowl and mix at low speed to blend well. Beat water, eggs, oil, and vanilla together with a fork or small whip until well blended, and then add to flour mixture. Beat together at medium speed only until smooth. Spread batter evenly in a 9-inch square cake pan that has been sprayed with pan spray or greased with margarine.

Bake at 350°F for 30 to 35 minutes, or until cake pulls away from the sides of the pan and a cake tester comes out clean from the center. Cool on a wire rack. Cut four by four.

Yield: 16 servings
Food exchanges per serving: 1 starch and 1 fat; or 1 carbohydrate choice
Sugar per serving: 1 teaspoon or 4 grams
Low-cholesterol diets: Omit eggs. Use ½ cup egg whites or liquid egg substitute.
Low-sodium diets: Omit salt. Use low-sodium baking powder.
Nutritive values per serving:

Calories: 119	FAT: 6 g
CHO: 15 g	Na: 120 mg
PRO: 3 g	Cholesterol: 34 mg

Cassata

This cake has always been a favorite of mine because it is so easy to make and keeps beautifully for a couple of days. Italian families use it for festive occasions and it always reminds me of times in the past when we have served it for special meals.

1¼ cups cake flour
1 teaspoon baking powder
¼ teaspoon salt
1 cup (5 to 6 medium) eggs
¼ cup sugar
½ teaspoon cream of tartar
¼ cup water at room
   temperature
2 teaspoons vanilla extract
1 pound part-skim ricotta
   cheese

2 tablespoons chopped candied
   cherries
3 tablespoons miniature
   chocolate chips
1 tablespoon raisins
10 1-gram packets Equal sugar
   substitute
2 to 3 tablespoons orange
   liqueur or orange juice
1 tablespoon powdered
   sugar

Stir cake flour, baking powder, and salt together to blend well and set aside.

Place eggs in mixer bowl and mix at medium speed until thick and lemon colored. Add sugar and cream of tartar to eggs and beat at high speed, using a whip, for 10 minutes. Combine water and vanilla and add slowly to egg mixture while beating at low speed. Add flour mixture while continuing to beat at low speed. Do not overmix. Spread half of the batter evenly in each of two 9-inch-layer cake pans that have been greased, lined with wax paper on the bottom, and then the bottom greased again. (Do not grease the sides of the pan or line them with wax paper.)

Bake at 375°F for about 15 minutes, or until the layers are lightly browned and spring back when touched in the center. Turn the layers out onto a wire rack, remove the wax paper immediately, and cool to room temperature.

Drain any excess liquid from the ricotta, but do not press out any liquid. Discard the liquid and place the cheese in a small bowl. Add the cherries, chocolate chips, raisins, sugar substitute, and orange liqueur or orange juice and mix lightly. The mixture should be soft but hold its shape. Place a cake layer on a plate and spread the cheese mixture evenly on top of the cake layer. Cover with the second layer.

Wrap in aluminum foil and refrigerate overnight or up to 2 or 3 days, if desired.

Remove the cake from the refrigerator, sprinkle evenly with powdered sugar, and cut into 16 equal pieces.

Yield: 16 (1-slice) servings
Food exchanges per serving: 1 starch and 1 meat; or 1 carbohydrate
   choice
Sugar per serving: 2.1 teaspoons or 9 grams
Low-cholesterol diets: Liquid egg substitute does not work well in this
   recipe. Use your own discretion for inclusion in your diet.
Low-sodium diets: Omit salt. Use low-sodium baking powder.
Nutritive values per serving:

Calories: 133	FAT: 5 g
CHO: 16 g	Na: 111 mg
PRO: 6 g	Cholesterol: 17 mg

Cherry Cheesecake

This is a good cake to take along to a potluck luncheon or dinner. It looks pretty, tastes good, and provides a dessert you can eat with a clear conscience.

Cherry Topping

1¾ cups (16-ounce can) unsweetened red pitted cherries
1 tablespoon cornstarch

¼ teaspoon almond extract
12 1-gram packets Equal sugar substitute or another sugar substitute

Crust

12 2¼-inch graham crackers

3 tablespoons sugar
¼ cup margarine, melted

Filling

3 packets (2½ tablespoons) plain gelatin
2 tablespoons sugar
1½ cups boiling water
12 1-gram packets Equal sugar substitute or another sugar substitute

⅓ cup lemon juice
2 pounds part-skim ricotta cheese
2 teaspoons vanilla extract
½ teaspoon salt
12 1-gram packets Equal or another sugar substitute

For topping: Drain cherries well, reserving the juice. Add water to the juice, if necessary, to make 1 cup liquid. Set the cherries aside and mix the juice with the cornstarch, stirring until smooth. Cook and stir over moderate heat until mixture is clear and thickened and the starchy taste is gone. Remove from the heat, add almond extract, 12 packets of sugar substitute, and cherries and refrigerate until needed.

For crust: Crush the graham crackers and place in a 9 × 13-inch cake pan along with 3 tablespoons sugar and melted margarine. Mix with your fingers to blend well and then pat evenly in the bottom of the pan and set aside until needed.

For filling: Stir the gelatin and 2 tablespoons sugar together to blend well, add the boiling water, and stir until the gelatin is dissolved. Add 12 packets of sugar substitute and lemon juice and set aside a few minutes until it begins to thicken.

Drain any excess liquid from the cheese but do not press it to remove any further liquid. Place the cheese in a bowl along with the vanilla, salt, and 12 packets of sugar substitute. Mix lightly until smooth. Add the gelatin mixture, which should be syrupy, and mix until smooth.

Pour the cheese mixture over the graham cracker crust and refrigerate until thickened. Spread the cherry mixture evenly over the filling.

Cut into 18 equal squares. Use 1 square per serving.

Note: Other types of sugar substitute may be used, if desired, using sugar substitute equal to ½ cup sugar for each 12 packets of Equal. I have used Equal here because I prefer the taste of it.

Yield: 18 servings
Food exchanges per serving: 1 milk and 1 fat; or 1 carbohydrate
    choice
Sugar per serving: .5 teaspoon or 2 grams
Low-cholesterol diets: Recipe is suitable as written.
Low-sodium diets: Omit salt.
Nutritive values per serving:

Calories: 146	FAT: 7 g
CHO: 13 g	Na: 418 mg
PRO: 7 g	Cholesterol: 3 mg

Chocolate Kraut Cake

You can't taste the sauerkraut in this cake. It tastes like a good chocolate coconut cake; my sister says it reminds her of her favorite candy bar.

½ cup (1 stick) margarine
½ cup sugar
Dry sugar substitute equal to ½ cup sugar
1½ teaspoons coconut flavoring
2 large eggs
2 cups all-purpose flour
½ cup unsweetened cocoa powder
1 teaspoon baking soda
1 teaspoon baking powder
1 cup water at room temperature
⅔ cup drained, chopped sauerkraut

Cream margarine, sugar, and dry sugar substitute together at medium speed until light and fluffy. Add flavoring and eggs, and mix at medium speed for 30 seconds, scraping down the bowl before and after adding eggs. Stir flour, cocoa, baking soda and baking powder together to blend well. Add, along with water, to creamed mixture and mix at medium speed until smooth and creamy. Add sauerkraut and mix lightly. Spread batter evenly in a 9 × 13-inch cake pan that has been sprayed with pan spray or greased with margarine.

Bake at 375°F for 30 to 35 minutes, or until cake pulls away from the sides of the pan and a cake tester comes out clean from the center. Cool on a wire rack to room temperature. Cut three by six.

Yield: 18 servings
Food exchanges per serving: 1 starch and 1 fat; or 1 carbohydrate choice
Sugar per serving: 1.3 teaspoons or 5 grams
Low-cholesterol diets: Omit eggs. Use ½ cup egg whites or liquid egg substitute.
Low-sodium diets: Use salt-free margarine and low-sodium baking powder.
Nutritive values per serving:

Calories: 134
CHO: 18 g
PRO: 3 g
FAT: 6 g
Na: 188 mg
Cholesterol: 30 mg

Chocolate Oat Bran Cake

Don't let the thought of oat bran stop you from trying this cake. It is delicious, and most people never guess it is diabetic or contains oat bran.

1 cup oat bran cereal
1 cup water
1 large egg
⅓ cup vegetable oil
Dry sugar substitute equal to ⅓ cup sugar
1 teaspoon vanilla extract
1 teaspoon chocolate flavoring (optional)

1 tablespoon white vinegar
1 cup all-purpose flour
⅓ cup sugar
¼ cup unsweetened cocoa powder
2 tablespoons instant dry milk
1 teaspoon baking soda
½ teaspoon cinnamon
½ teaspoon salt

Place cereal, water, egg, oil, dry sugar substitute, flavorings, and vinegar in a mixer bowl. Mix lightly and let stand for 30 to 45 minutes. (This timing is very important.)

Stir flour, sugar, cocoa, dry milk, baking soda, cinnamon, and salt together to blend well. Add to cereal mixture and mix at medium speed about 1 minute, or until well blended. Spread batter evenly in a 9-inch square cake pan that has been sprayed with pan spray or greased with margarine.

Bake at 350°F for about 35 minutes, or until cake pulls away from the sides of the pan and a cake tester comes out clean from the center. Cool on a wire rack. Cut four by four.

Yield: 16 servings
Food exchanges per serving: 1 starch and 1 fat; or 1 carbohydrate choice
Sugar per serving: 1 teaspoon or 4 grams
Low-cholesterol diets: Omit egg. Use ¼ cup egg whites or liquid egg substitute.
Low-sodium diets: Omit salt.
Nutritive values per serving:

Calories: 114   FAT: 6 g
CHO: 15 g   Na: 126 mg
PRO: 2 g   Cholesterol: 17 mg

Chocolate Sponge Cake

1 1/3 cups eggs at room
  temperature
1/2 cup sugar
1/4 cup all-purpose flour
1/4 cup unsweetened cocoa
  powder
1 teaspoon baking powder
1/2 teaspoon salt

Dry sugar substitute equal to 1/2
  cup sugar
1 teaspoon vanilla extract
1 teaspoon chocolate flavoring
  (optional)
3 tablespoons vegetable oil
2 tablespoons powdered sugar

Place eggs and sugar in a mixer bowl and mix at high speed, using a whip, until mixture holds a crease when you remove the whip. Stir flour, cocoa, baking powder, salt, and dry sugar substitute together to blend well. Add flour mixture slowly to egg mixture while whipping at slow speed. When the flour is almost absorbed, slowly pour flavorings and oil into mixture, beating at slow speed. Pour batter into a 9 × 13-inch cake pan that has been sprayed with pan spray or greased with margarine, lined with wax paper (which should hang over the pan a little), and then greased again.

Bake at 350°F for 25 to 30 minutes, or until cake springs back when touched in the center. Turn cake out onto a wire rack immediately, removing the wax paper right away if you have used it. Sprinkle with powdered sugar. Cool to room temperature. Cut three by four.

Yield: 12 servings
Food exchanges per serving: 1 starch and 1 fat; or 1 carbohydrate
  choice
Sugar per serving: 2 teaspoons or 8 grams
Low-cholesterol diets: Recipe is not suitable.
Low-sodium diets: Omit salt.
Nutritive values per serving:

Calories: 128	FAT: 6 g
CHO: 15 g	Na: 145 mg
PRO: 4 g	Cholesterol: 114 mg

Dark Chocolate Cake

This rich, dark cake tastes as if it were made with lots of melted chocolate.

1¾ cups all-purpose flour
⅓ cup sugar
Dry sugar substitute equal to ½ cup sugar
½ cup unsweetened cocoa powder
2 tablespoons instant dry milk
1 teaspoon baking soda

1 teaspoon baking powder
¼ cup water at room temperature
½ cup egg whites
⅓ cup vegetable oil
2 teaspoons vanilla extract
¾ cup boiling-hot water

Place flour, sugar, dry sugar substitute, cocoa, dry milk, baking soda, and baking powder in a mixer bowl and mix at low speed to blend well. Combine room-temperature water, egg whites, oil, and vanilla, and mix well with a fork. Add, along with boiling-hot water, to flour mixture, and mix at medium speed for 2 minutes. Pour batter into a 9 × 13-inch pan that has been sprayed with pan spray or greased with margarine.

Bake at 375°F for 30 to 35 minutes, or until cake pulls away from the sides of the pan and a cake tester comes out clean from the center. Cool on a wire rack. Cut four by four.

Yield: 16 servings
Food exchanges per serving: 1 starch and 1 fat; or 1 carbohydrate choice
Sugar per serving: 1 teaspoon or 4 grams
Low-cholesterol diets: Recipe is suitable as written.
Low-sodium diets: Use low-sodium baking powder.
Nutritive values per serving:

Calories: 118
CHO: 16 g
PRO: 3 g
FAT: 5 g
Na: 88 mg
Cholesterol: 0

Dundee Cake

This English cake is traditionally cut in thin slices and served with tea or lemonade. It is available in most stores and bakeries in England, although not in this lower sugar version. I like it because it reminds me of having tea in England and also because it is just plain good. I made it once for a woman who moved in next door and she complimented me on my good fruit bread, so I'll let you judge whether you think it is a good bread or cake.

¼ cup (½ stick) margarine	½ teaspoon allspice
⅓ cup sugar	½ teaspoon nutmeg
1 cup (5 to 6 medium) eggs at room temperature	½ teaspoon cinnamon
1½ cups all-purpose flour	¼ cup raisins
2 teaspoons baking powder	¼ cup chopped pecans
	2 tablespoons chopped candied cherries

Cream margarine and sugar together in a mixer bowl at medium speed until light and fluffy. Add eggs and beat at medium speed to blend well. Scrape down the bowl. Stir flour, baking powder, allspice, nutmeg, and cinnamon together to blend well.

Add flour mixture to creamed mixture and beat at medium speed about 30 seconds, or until blended. Add raisins, nuts, and cherries to the batter and mix lightly.

Spread the batter evenly in a 9 × 5-inch loaf pan that has been sprayed with pan spray or well greased with margarine.

Bake at 350°F for about 45 minutes, or until a cake tester comes out clean from the center of the cake and the cake starts to pull away from the sides of the pan. Cool 10 minutes in the pan and then turn out onto a wire rack to cool to room temperature. Cut into 18 equal slices, about ½ inch thick, and use 1 slice per serving.

Yield: 18 servings

Food exchanges per serving: 1 starch and 1 fat; or 1 carbohydrate choice

Sugar per serving: .9 teaspoon or 3.7 grams

Low-cholesterol diets: Omit eggs. Use 1 cup liquid egg substitute.

Low-sodium diets: Omit salt. Use salt-free margarine and low-sodium baking powder.

Nutritive values per serving:

Calories: 118	FAT: 5 g
CHO: 15 g	Na: 86 mg
PRO: 3 g	Cholesterol: 47 mg

Mocha Nut Cake

I once took this cake over to my friend Vera Wilson's. She had unexpected company, and we all had a good time visiting—and eating the cake.

3/4 cup very hot water
1 tablespoon freeze-dried coffee
1/2 cup (1 stick) margarine
1/3 cup brown sugar
Dry sugar substitute equal to 1/2 cup sugar
1 large egg
1 teaspoon vanilla extract

1 1/2 cups all-purpose flour
1/3 cup unsweetened cocoa powder
2 tablespoons instant nonfat dry milk
2 teaspoons baking powder
1/4 teaspoon salt
1/4 cup chopped nuts

Combine hot water and freeze-dried coffee, and set aside for later use. Cream margarine, brown sugar, and dry sugar substitute together at medium speed until light and fluffy. Add egg and vanilla, and mix at medium speed for 1 minute, scraping down the bowl before and after adding egg and vanilla. Stir flour, cocoa, dry milk, baking powder, and salt together to blend. Add, along with coffee and nuts, to creamed mixture. Mix at medium speed until batter is smooth. Spread batter evenly in a 9-inch square cake pan that has been sprayed with pan spray or greased with margarine.

Bake at 350°F for about 30 minutes, or until cake pulls away from the sides of the pan and a cake tester comes out clean from the center. Cool on a wire rack. Cut four by four.

Yield: 16 servings
Food exchanges per serving: 1 starch and 1 1/2 fat; or 1 carbohydrate choice
Sugar per serving: 1 teaspoon or 4 grams
Low-cholesterol diets: Omit egg. Use 1/4 cup egg whites or liquid egg substitute.
Low-sodium diets: Omit salt. Use low-sodium baking powder.
Nutritive values per serving:

Calories: 135
CHO: 15 g
PRO: 2 g

FAT: 8 g
Na: 151 mg
Cholesterol: 17 mg

Brownie Cupcakes

These cupcakes earned their name because their taste and texture remind me of brownies. They are a dark, rich chocolate, and I think they are luscious.

1¼ cups all-purpose flour
¼ cup sugar
Dry sugar substitute equal to ½ cup sugar
½ cup unsweetened cocoa powder
2 tablespoons instant dry milk

1 teaspoon baking powder
½ teaspoon salt
½ teaspoon cinnamon
¼ cup water
⅓ cup vegetable oil
2 large eggs
2 teaspoons vanilla extract

Place flour, sugar, dry sugar substitute, cocoa, dry milk, baking powder, salt, and cinnamon in a mixer bowl and mix at low speed to blend well. Beat water, oil, eggs, and vanilla together with a fork to blend, and then add to flour mixture. Mix at medium speed until batter is shiny. Fill a 12-muffin pan that has been sprayed with pan spray, lined with paper liners, or greased with margarine, about half full (about 2½ tablespoons per cupcake).

Bake at 350°F for 20 to 25 minutes, or until a cake tester comes out clean from the center of a cupcake. *Do not overbake.* Remove cupcakes from pan and cool on a wire rack.

Yield: 12 servings
Food exchanges per serving: 1 starch and 1½ fat; or 1 carbohydrate choice
Sugar per serving: 1 teaspoon or 4 grams
Low-cholesterol diets: Omit eggs. Use ½ cup egg whites or liquid egg substitute.
Low-sodium diets: Omit salt. Use low-sodium baking powder.
Nutritive values per serving:

Calories: 142
CHO: 17 g
PRO: 3 g

FAT: 8 g
Na: 132 mg
Cholesterol: 46 mg

Banana Nut Cake

My friend Jean Fenner kept asking me when I would have a banana cake appropriate for diabetics; developing one was a sort of a challenge. I came up with this, which suits me and, I hope, Jean too.

⅓ cup (⅔ stick) margarine	1¾ cups all-purpose flour
⅓ cup sugar	1 teaspoon baking powder
Sugar substitute equal to ½ cup sugar	½ teaspoon baking soda
	½ teaspoon salt
2 large eggs	1 cup mashed bananas
1 teaspoon vanilla extract	¼ cup chopped English walnuts

Cream margarine, sugar, and sugar substitute together at medium speed until light and fluffy. Add eggs and vanilla, and mix at medium speed until creamy, scraping down the bowl before and after adding eggs and vanilla. Stir flour, baking powder, baking soda, and salt together to blend well, and add to creamed mixture along with bananas and walnuts. Mix at medium speed until creamy. Spread batter evenly in a 9-inch square cake pan that has been sprayed with pan spray or greased with margarine.

Bake at 350°F for 30 to 35 minutes, or until cake pulls away from the sides of the pan and a cake tester comes out clean from the center. Cool on a wire rack to room temperature. Cut four by four.

Yield: 16 servings

Food exchanges per serving: 1 starch and 1 fat; or 1 carbohydrate choice

Sugar per serving: 1 teaspoon or 4 grams

Low-cholesterol diets: Omit eggs. Use ½ cup egg whites or liquid egg substitute.

Low-sodium diets: Omit salt. Use low-sodium baking powder and salt-free margarine.

Nutritive values per serving:

Calories: 121	FAT: 6 g
CHO: 15 g	Na: 166 mg
PRO: 3 g	Cholesterol: 34 mg

Genoise

This French cake, which Frances Nielsen taught me to make, is a perfect basis for fruit shortcakes. Jan's mother, Boots Jorgensen, says this is what she thinks of when she wants strawberry shortcake, not the baking-powder biscuits common in the Midwest. Boots's husband, Leon, has diabetes. She can serve him shortcake using this cake and strawberries sweetened with Equal sugar substitute.

1/4 cup (1/2 stick) margarine
1 1/4 cups (7 to 8 medium) eggs
   at room temperature
1/2 cup sugar
1 teaspoon almond or lemon
   flavoring

1 cup all-purpose flour
1 teaspoon baking powder
1/2 teaspoon salt
Dry sugar substitute equal
   to 1/3 cup sugar
   (optional)

Melt margarine and set aside to cool to room temperature. Grease a 9 × 13-inch cake pan well with margarine or pan spray. Cut a piece of 12-inch-wide wax paper 15 inches long. Line the pan evenly with the paper, letting it extend up ends and sides of the pan. Grease the wax paper again with margarine or spray lightly, and set aside for later use.

Place eggs and sugar in a mixing bowl, and beat, using a whip, at high speed for several minutes, or until mixture holds a crease when the beater is withdrawn. Beat in flavoring.

Stir flour, baking powder, salt, and sugar substitute (if using) together to blend well. Add flour mixture to egg mixture 1/4 cup at a time and beat at low speed until partially blended. Pour margarine slowly into batter while beating at low speed. Pour batter into prepared pan and smooth the top of the batter evenly with a spatula, if necessary.

Bake at 350°F for 25 to 30 minutes, or until cake is lightly browned and springs back when touched in the center. Turn out onto a wire rack and remove the wax paper immediately. Cool to room temperature and cut into 12 equal pieces.

Yield: 12 squares
Food exchanges per serving: 1 starch and 1 1/2 fat; or 1 carbohydrate
   choice
Sugar per serving: 2 teaspoons or 8 grams
Low-cholesterol diets: Liquid egg substitute is not suitable in this type
   of cake. Use your own discretion for inclusion in your diet.
Low-sodium diets: Omit salt. Use low-sodium baking powder.
Nutritive values per serving:

Calories: 100
CHO: 12 g
PRO: 1 g

FAT: 5 g
Na: 40 mg
Cholesterol: 5 mg

Gingerbread

This dark, rich gingerbread is almost like a cake. If you prefer a more pronounced ginger flavor, use 2 teaspoons ginger and no cinnamon.

½ cup (1 stick) margarine
½ cup molasses
⅓ cup egg whites
2 cups all-purpose flour
1 teaspoon baking powder
1 teaspoon baking soda

1 teaspoon ginger
1 teaspoon cinnamon
½ teaspoon salt
Dry sugar substitute equal to
  ½ cup sugar
¾ cup very hot water

Cream margarine and molasses together at medium speed until light and fluffy. Add egg whites and mix at medium speed 30 seconds, scraping down the bowl before and after adding egg whites. Stir flour, baking powder, baking soda, ginger, cinnamon, salt, and dry sugar substitute together to blend well. Add, along with water, to creamed mixture. Mix at medium speed only until smooth. Pour batter into a 9-inch square cake pan that has been sprayed with pan spray or greased with margarine.

Bake at 375°F for 35 to 40 minutes, or until gingerbread pulls away from the sides of the pan and a cake tester comes out clean from the center. Cool on a wire rack. Cut four by four.

Yield: 16 servings
Food exchanges per serving: 1 starch and 1 fat; or 1 carbohydrate choice
Sugar per serving: 1.5 teaspoons or 6 grams
Low-cholesterol diets: Recipe is suitable as written.
Low-sodium diets: Omit salt. Use salt-free margarine and low-sodium baking powder.
Nutritive values per serving:

Calories: 132
CHO: 18 g
PRO: 2 g

FAT: 6 g
Na: 224 mg
Cholesterol: 0

Honey Cake

This recipe is based on one for a Jewish honey cake from my friend Anita Kane, of Milwaukee, who has given me many wonderful recipes. Anita is diabetic also, so she is always interested in good diabetic recipes.

1/4 cup sugar
1/4 cup honey
1/3 cup vegetable oil
2 large eggs
2 teaspoons vanilla extract
Dry sugar substitute equal to
    1/3 cup sugar

2 cups all-purpose flour
2 teaspoons baking powder
1/2 teaspoon baking soda
1/4 teaspoon salt
1 1/2 tablespoons instant
    coffee
3/4 cup boiling-hot water

Place sugar, honey, oil, eggs, vanilla, and dry sugar substitute in a bowl and mix at medium speed to blend well. Stir flour, baking powder, baking soda, and salt together to blend well. Add coffee to water, mix, and add, along with flour mixture, to creamy mixture. Mix at medium speed only until creamy. Spread batter evenly in a 9 × 5-inch loaf pan that has been sprayed with pan spray or greased with margarine.

Bake at 375°F for about 45 minutes, or until cake pulls away from the sides of the pan and a cake tester comes out clean from the center. Remove pan to a wire rack and cool for 10 minutes; then turn cake out onto the rack and cool to room temperature. Cut into 18 equal slices 1/2 inch thick.

Yield: 18 servings
Food exchanges per serving: 1 starch and 1 fat; or 1 carbohydrate choice
Sugar per serving: 1.3 teaspoons or 5 grams
Low-cholesterol diets: Omit eggs. Use 1/2 cup liquid egg substitute.
Low-sodium diets: Omit salt. Use low-sodium baking powder.
Nutritive values per serving:

Calories: 119
CHO: 17 g
PRO: 2 g

FAT: 5 g
Na: 97 mg
Cholesterol: 30 mg

Lemon Cake

This cake has a light, delicate flavor. It is good plain or served with whipped diabetic topping flavored with lemon.

2 cups all-purpose flour
2 teaspoons baking powder
2 tablespoons instant nonfat
   dry milk
¼ cup sugar
Dry sugar substitute equal to
   ⅓ cup sugar
¼ teaspoon salt

1 cup water at room
   temperature
2 large eggs
⅓ cup vegetable oil
1 teaspoon lemon flavoring
1 tablespoon grated fresh or
   finely chopped dried lemon
   rind

Place flour, baking powder, dry milk, sugar, dry sugar substitute, and salt in a mixer bowl and mix 30 seconds at low speed to blend well. Beat water, eggs, oil, flavoring, and rind together with a fork to blend, and add to flour mixture. Mix at medium speed until creamy. Spread batter evenly in a 9-inch square cake pan that has been sprayed with pan spray or greased with margarine.

Bake at 350°F for 30 to 35 minutes, or until cake edges are lightly browned and a cake tester comes out clean from the center. Remove to a wire rack and cool to room temperature. Cut four by four.

Yield: 16 servings
Food exchanges per serving: 1 starch and 1 fat; or 1 carbohydrate
   choice
Sugar per serving: .8 teaspoon or 3 grams
Low-cholesterol diets: Omit eggs. Use ½ cup egg whites or liquid egg
   substitute.
Low-sodium diets: Omit salt. Use low-sodium baking powder.
Nutritive values per serving:

Calories: 131	FAT: 6 g
CHO: 16 g	Na: 87 mg
PRO: 3 g	Cholesterol: 34 mg

Lemon Buttermilk Cake

You can make this cake without the lemon rind, but it is better if you include it.

1/2 cup (1 stick) margarine
1/3 cup sugar
Dry sugar substitute equal to 1/3 cup sugar
1 1/2 teaspoons lemon flavoring
Grated rind of 1 lemon
2 large eggs

2 cups all-purpose flour
1 tablespoon dry buttermilk
1 teaspoon baking powder
1/2 teaspoon baking soda
1/4 teaspoon salt
3/4 cup water at room temperature

Place margarine, sugar, and dry sugar substitute in a mixer bowl and mix at medium speed until light and fluffy. Add flavoring, rind, and eggs, and mix at medium speed for 30 seconds, scraping down the bowl before and after adding them. Stir flour, dry buttermilk, baking powder, baking soda, and salt together, and add to mixture along with water. Beat at medium speed for 1 minute. Spread batter evenly in a 9-inch square cake pan that has been sprayed with pan spray or greased with margarine.

Bake at 350°F for 30 to 35 minutes, or until cake is lightly browned and a cake tester comes out clean from the center. Cool on a wire rack. Cut four by four.

Yield: 16 servings
Food exchanges per serving: 1 starch and 1 fat; or 1 carbohydrate choice
Sugar per serving: 1 teaspoon or 4 grams
Low-cholesterol diets: Omit eggs. Use 1/2 cup egg whites or liquid egg substitute.
Low-sodium diets: Omit salt. Use salt-free margarine.
Nutritive values per serving:

Calories: 135
CHO: 16 g
PRO: 3 g

FAT: 7 g
Na: 158 mg
Cholesterol: 35 mg

Lemon Cheesecake

Everyone loves cheesecake, but most such cakes are so high in calories and cholesterol that I don't make them. This one, however, is lighter and fits into my diet, so I make it for myself and others also.

3/4 cup graham cracker crumbs (8 crackers)

2 tablespoons margarine, melted

0.3-ounce package sugar-free lemon gelatin

1 cup boiling water

15 ounces part-skim ricotta cheese

8 ounces Neufchâtel (light cream) cheese

1 1/2 teaspoons lemon flavoring

3/4 cup powdered sugar

Stir graham cracker crumbs and margarine together to blend well. Set 2 tablespoons of mixture aside. Spread the rest of it evenly over the bottom of an 8-inch square cake pan. Bake at 350°F for 6 minutes, and then place pan on a wire rack to cool to room temperature.

Stir gelatin into water to dissolve the gelatin; refrigerate until gelatin is syrupy. Place ricotta (drain if necessary), Neufchâtel cheese, flavoring, and powdered sugar in a mixer bowl and mix at medium speed until smooth. Add gelatin to cheese mixture and mix at medium speed to blend. Pour cheese mixture on top of baked crust and sprinkle reserved crumbs over cheese layer. Refrigerate until firm. Cut three by four.

Variation: Strawberry Cheesecake: Use sugar-free strawberry gelatin instead of lemon gelatin. Use all of crumb mixture for bottom crust and garnish each serving with a fresh strawberry.

Yield: 12 servings

Food exchanges per serving: 1 starch and 1 fat; or 1 carbohydrate choice

Sugar per serving: 1.5 teaspoons or 6 grams

Low-cholesterol diets: Recipe is suitable as written.

Low-sodium diets: Use salt-free margarine.

Nutritive values per serving:

Calories: 173

CHO: 17 g

PRO: 10 g

FAT: 7 g

Na: 277 mg

Cholesterol: 28 mg

Madeira Cake

This is a rather rich but plain, unfrosted English cake. There is no Madeira wine in it; it is called Madeira cake because it is often served, unfrosted, with Madeira wine.

½ cup (1 stick) margarine
½ cup sugar
Dry sugar substitute equal to ½ cup sugar
2 teaspoons lemon flavoring

4 large eggs
1¾ cups all-purpose flour
1½ teaspoons baking powder
½ teaspoon salt

Cream margarine, sugar, dry sugar substitute, and flavoring together at medium speed until light and fluffy. Add eggs, one at a time, beating well after each addition, scraping down the bowl before and after adding eggs. Stir flour, baking powder, and salt together and add to egg mixture. Mix at medium speed only until creamy. Spread batter evenly in a 9 × 5-inch loaf pan that has been sprayed with pan spray or greased well with margarine.

Bake at 350°F for about 1 hour, or until cake is lightly browned and a cake tester comes out clean from the center. Remove pan to a wire rack and let cool for 10 minutes; then turn cake out onto the rack and cool to room temperature. Cut into 18 equal slices ½ inch wide.

Yield: 18 servings
Food exchanges per serving: 1 starch and 1 fat; or 1 carbohydrate choice
Sugar per serving: 1.3 teaspoons or 5.5 grams
Low-cholesterol diets: Recipe is not suitable. Liquid egg substitute does not yield a good cake.
Low-sodium diets: Omit salt. Use salt-free margarine and low-sodium baking powder.
Nutritive values per serving:

Calories: 129
CHO: 15 g
PRO: 3 g

FAT: 7 g
Na: 142 mg
Cholesterol: 56 mg

Orange Licorice Cake

If you have fond memories of long black licorice sticks, you will like this cake. If you don't like licorice, omit the anise seed and you'll have a good plain orange cake.

1¾ cups all-purpose
   flour
¼ cup dry orange-flavored
   breakfast drink mix (not
   sugar-free)
2 tablespoons sugar
2 tablespoons instant
   nonfat dry milk

½ teaspoon baking soda
1 tablespoon anise seed
½ teaspoon salt
½ cup (1 stick) margarine at
   room temperature
1 large egg
¾ cup water at room
   temperature

Place flour, drink mix, sugar, dry milk, baking soda, anise seed, and salt in a mixer bowl and mix at low speed to blend well. Add margarine, egg, and water, and mix at medium speed until smooth. Spread batter evenly in a 9-inch square cake pan that has been sprayed with pan spray or greased with margarine.

Bake at 350°F for about 35 minutes, or until cake is lightly browned and pulls away from the sides of the pan and a cake tester comes out clean from the center. Cool on a wire rack to room temperature. Cut four by four.

Yield: 16 servings
Food exchanges per serving: 1 starch and 1 fat; or 1 carbohydrate
   choice
Sugar per serving: 1.1 teaspoons or 4.5 grams
Low-cholesterol diets: Omit egg. Use ¼ cup egg whites or liquid egg
   substitute.
Low-sodium diets: Omit salt. Use salt-free margarine.
Nutritive values per serving:

Calories: 151
CHO: 15 g
PRO: 2 g

FAT: 6 g
Na: 223 mg
Cholesterol: 16 mg

Petits Fours

I call these petits fours because they are small and decorative, and look very pretty on a platter.

16-ounce package
   commercial angel food
   cake mix

1 cup (6 ounces) semisweet
   chocolate chips
½ cup chopped nuts

Prepare an 11 × 15-inch jelly roll pan by washing it well with soap and water, drying it and then lining the bottom of the pan with aluminum foil. (Smooth the foil carefully so the cake will be even.)

Prepare cake mix as directed on the package. Spread batter evenly in the jelly roll pan and bake at 350°F for about 25 minutes, or until cake is lightly browned and the center springs back when touched. Turn cake out onto a wire rack, remove the aluminum foil, and cool to room temperature. Refrigerate cake on the wire rack for 30 minutes, to make cake firmer.

Melt chocolate chips, add nuts, and spread mixture evenly over top of cake. Mark cake four by seven: with a knife, draw lines through the chocolate but not through cake. Return cake to the refrigerator to firm up chocolate. When it is chilled and firm, cut through cake on the marked lines with a sharp serrated knife.

Note: If you want to freeze the cake, freeze it without the chocolate. Add the chocolate before you serve the cake, allowing time for the chocolate mixture to become firm.

Yield: 28 servings
Food exchanges per serving: 1 starch and 1 fat; or 1 carbohydrate
   choice
Sugar per serving: 1.9 teaspoons or 8 grams
Low-cholesterol diets: Recipe is suitable as written.
Low-sodium diets: Recipe is suitable as written.
Nutritive values per serving:

Calories: 101
CHO: 17 g
PRO: 2 g

FAT: 4 g
Na: 67 mg
Cholesterol: 0

Swiss Chocolate Roll

Chocolate lovers can enjoy this tasty dessert without having to budget a lot of carbohydrates. The roll uses a combination of bananas, bread, and ricotta cheese to replace traditional fats and sugars. Best yet, it's easy to make and elegant to serve.

- 1 medium-size ripe banana
- 2 large eggs
- 2 slices white bread, with crusts
- 2/3 cup instant nonfat dry milk
- 4 teaspoons unsweetened cocoa powder

- 2 teaspoons vanilla extract
- 1/2 teaspoon almond extract
- 1 teaspoon cream of tartar
- 1 teaspoon baking powder
- 1 teaspoon soda
- Dry sugar substitute equal to 4 teaspoons sugar

Filling

- 2/3 cup part-skim ricotta cheese
- 1 1/2 teaspoons vanilla
- Dry sugar substitute equal to 4 teaspoons sugar

- Powdered sugar for dusting (optional)

Line an 8-inch square pan with wax paper; spray the top of the paper well with cooking spray. Process all ingredients (except filling) in a blender, adding small amounts at a time, until smooth. Pour the batter in the pan.

Bake at 325°F for 10 to 12 minutes. Cool slightly. Remove cake from pan while warm and roll like a jelly roll. Wrap the cake roll in the wax paper and cool completely. Meanwhile, prepare the filling.

For filling: Blend all filling ingredients together in a clean blender until smooth. Unroll cooled cake and spread mixture evenly over it. Roll cake again into jelly roll. Chill until completely cool. Dust lightly with powdered sugar if using. Cut roll into 8 1-inch slices.

Yield: 8 servings
Food exchanges per serving: 1 starch and 1/2 fat; or 1 carbohydrate choice
Sugar per serving: 1.4 teaspoons or 6 grams
Low-cholesterol diets: Recipe is suitable as written.
Low-sodium diets: Use your own discretion for inclusion in your diet.
Nutritive values per serving:

Calories: 103	FAT: 3 g
CHO: 12 g	Na: 263 mg
PRO: 7 g	Cholesterol: 60 mg

Pumpkin Roll

This cake freezes well, so it can be prepared ahead of time. To thaw it, put it in the refrigerator in its foil wrapping.

Filling

¼ cup powdered sugar
⅓ cup Sugar Twin dry sugar substitute, plus additional for sprinkling

4 ounces Neufchâtel (light cream) cheese
8 ounces well-drained part-skim ricotta cheese
1 teaspoon lemon juice

Cake

¾ cup all-purpose flour
1 tablespoon pumpkin pie spice
1 teaspoon baking soda
1 teaspoon baking powder
3 large eggs

½ cup granulated sugar
1 teaspoon lemon juice
⅔ cup canned solid pack pumpkin

For filling: Combine powdered sugar, dry sugar substitute, and Neufchâtel cheese, and mix until smooth. Add ricotta cheese and lemon juice, and mix only to blend. Set this filling aside for later use.

For cake: Stir flour, pumpkin pie spice, baking soda, and baking powder together to blend well. Set aside for later use.

Combine eggs and granulated sugar, and beat with a whip at high speed for about 5 minutes, or until thick and lemon colored. Add lemon juice, pumpkin, and flour mixture to egg mixture and mix at low speed, using the paddle, to blend well. Spread batter evenly in an 11 × 15-inch jelly roll pan that has been greased with margarine, lined with wax paper, and greased again, or that has a nonstick surface which has been sprayed with pan spray.

Bake at 375°F for 15 minutes, or until firm. Turn cake out onto a clean dishtowel sprinkled with Sugar Twin dry sugar substitute. Remove the wax paper, if used, as quickly as possible; roll cake in the dishtowel as you would a jelly roll. Cool to room temperature. Open the roll and spread evenly with cheese filling mixture. Roll cake again into a roll without the dishtowel, wrap in aluminum foil, and refrigerate for 4 hours, or until firm, or freeze to serve later. Cut into 16 equal slices.

Yield: 16 servings
Food exchanges per serving: 1 starch and 1 fat; or 1 carbohydrate
  choice
Sugar per serving: 1.9 teaspoons or 8 grams
Low-cholesterol diets: Recipe is not suitable.
Low-sodium diets: Use low-sodium baking powder.
Nutritive values per serving:

Calories: 115	FAT: 4 g
CHO: 15 g	Na: 127 mg
PRO: 5 g	Cholesterol: 54 mg

Ricotta Cheesecake

This recipe is based on one published by the makers of Sargento ricotta cheese, with my adaptations for a carbohydrate-controlled diet.

Crust

1 cup graham cracker
crumbs (11 or 12
crackers)
2 tablespoons sugar

Dry sugar substitute equal to
1/4 cup sugar
1/4 cup (1/2 stick) margarine,
melted

Filling

2 large eggs
1/4 cup half-and-half
2 tablespoons all-purpose flour
Dry sugar substitute equal to 1/2
cup sugar
1 tablespoon fresh lemon juice

1 tablespoon grated fresh or
finely chopped dried lemon
rind
1/4 teaspoon salt
15-ounce container low-fat
ricotta cheese

Topping

1 cup light sour cream
2 tablespoons sugar

1 teaspoon vanilla
extract

For crust: Place graham cracker crumbs, sugar, dry sugar substitute equal to 1/4 cup sugar, and margarine in an 8-inch square cake pan. Blend together with fingers and then spread evenly in the bottom and 1 1/2 inches up the sides of the pan. Refrigerate until needed.

For filling: Combine eggs, half-and-half, flour, dry sugar substitute equal to 1/2 cup sugar, lemon juice, lemon rind, and salt. Mix to blend well; add ricotta cheese and mix lightly to blend. Spread cheese mixture evenly over chilled crust. Bake at 350°F for 50 to 60 minutes, or until center is set.

For topping: Combine sour cream, sugar, and vanilla, and spread mixture evenly over filling. Return cheesecake to the oven for 10 minutes. Then turn off the oven, open the door, and leave cheesecake in the oven for another 40 minutes. Remove to a wire rack, cool to room temperature, and refrigerate until served. Cut three by three.

Yield: 9 servings

Food exchanges per serving: 1 milk, 1 vegetable, and 2 fat; or 1
carbohydrate choice

Sugar per serving: 1.3 teaspoons or 5 grams

Low-cholesterol diets: Recipe may be used at your discretion.

Low-sodium diets: Omit salt. Use salt-free margarine.

Nutritive values per serving:

Calories: 185	FAT: 12 g
CHO: 19 g	Na: 286 mg
PRO: 9 g	Cholesterol: 76 mg

White Cake

This special-occasion cake is good with a topping of unsweetened strawberries or other fresh fruit; it can also be frosted with diabetic frosting for a birthday or other special celebration. The recipe is based on one given to me by my friend Arlene Tapper White, who made many decorated wedding and birthday cakes as well as teaching and pursuing numerous activities including her church and Eastern Star group.

½ cup (1 stick) margarine at room temperature
½ cup sugar
Dry sugar substitute equal to ½ cup sugar
1 teaspoon vanilla extract
½ teaspoon almond extract (optional)

⅓ cup egg whites at room temperature
2 cups cake flour
2 teaspoons baking powder
2 tablespoons instant dry milk
½ cup water at room temperature

Cream margarine, sugar, dry sugar substitute, and flavorings together until light and fluffy. Add egg whites and mix together at medium speed for 1 minute, scraping down the bowl before and after adding egg whites. Stir flour, baking powder, and dry milk together to blend, and add, along with water, to creamed mixture. Mix at medium speed only until creamy. Spread batter evenly in a 9-inch square cake pan that has been sprayed with pan spray or greased with margarine.

Bake at 350°F for 30 to 35 minutes, or until cake is lightly browned and a cake tester comes out clean from the center. Cool on a wire rack. Cut four by four.

Yield: 16 servings
Food exchanges per serving: 1 starch and 1 fat; or 1 carbohydrate choice
Sugar per serving: 1.5 teaspoons or 6 grams
Low-cholesterol diets: Recipe is suitable as written.
Low-sodium diets: Use salt-free margarine and low-sodium baking powder.
Nutritive values per serving:

Calories: 124
CHO: 16 g
PRO: 2 g

FAT: 6 g
Na: 121 mg
Cholesterol: 0

White Loaf Cake

For the best results, all of the ingredients in this cake should be at room temperature, especially the margarine and egg whites. You may make the cake more festive by serving it with diabetic light whipped topping and a couple of fresh strawberries.

½ cup sugar
½ cup (1 stick) margarine
½ cup egg whites
1 teaspoon vanilla extract
1½ cups all-purpose flour

2 tablespoons instant nonfat dry milk
2 teaspoons baking powder
½ cup water

Cream sugar and margarine together at medium speed until light and fluffy. Add egg whites and vanilla, and mix at medium speed until creamy, scraping down the bowl before and after adding them. Stir flour, dry milk, and baking powder together to blend, and add, along with water, to creamy mixture. Mix at medium speed only until creamy. Spread batter evenly in a 9 × 5-inch loaf pan that has been sprayed with pan spray or greased with margarine.

Bake at 350°F for 45 to 50 minutes, or until cake is lightly browned and a cake tester comes out clean from the center. Let cake rest in the pan for 10 minutes; then turn cake out onto a wire rack and cool to room temperature. Cut into 16 equal slices ½ inch thick.

Yield: 16 servings
Food exchanges per serving: 1 starch and 1 fat; or 1 carbohydrate choice
Sugar per serving: 1.5 teaspoons or 6 grams
Low-cholesterol diets: Recipe is suitable as written.
Low-sodium diets: Use salt-free margarine and low-sodium baking powder.
Nutritive values per serving:

Calories: 123   FAT: 6 g
CHO: 16 g   Na: 123 mg
PRO: 2 g   Cholesterol: 0

Yellow Cake

2 cups cake flour
1/3 cup sugar
2 tablespoons dry buttermilk
Dry sugar substitute equal to 1/2
   cup sugar
1/2 teaspoon baking soda

1/2 teaspoon baking powder
1/4 cup water at room
   temperature
1/3 cup vegetable oil
3 large eggs
2 teaspoons vanilla extract

Place flour, sugar, dry buttermilk, dry sugar substitute, baking soda, and baking powder in a mixer bowl and mix at low speed to blend well. Beat water, oil, eggs, and vanilla together with a fork or small whip to blend well, and add to flour mixture. Mix at medium speed only until creamy. Pour batter into a 9-inch square cake pan that has been sprayed with pan spray or greased with margarine.

Bake at 375°F for 30 to 35 minutes, or until cake is lightly browned and pulls away from the sides of the pan and a cake tester comes out clean from the center. Cool on a wire rack. Cut four by four.

Note: Other flavorings, such as almond, lemon, or black walnut, may be used instead of vanilla.

Yield: 16 servings
Food exchanges per serving: 1 starch and 1 fat; or 1 carbohydrate
   choice
Sugar per serving: 1 teaspoon or 4 grams
Low-cholesterol diets: Omit eggs. Use 3/4 cup egg whites or liquid egg
   substitute.
Low-sodium diets: Use low-sodium baking powder.
Nutritive values per serving:

Calories: 118	FAT: 6 g
CHO: 14 g	Na: 54 mg
PRO: 2 g	Cholesterol: 52 mg

Butter Cream Frosting

I think this is the best diabetic frosting I've ever tasted.

½ cup water
2 tablespoons instant nonfat dry milk
2½ tablespoons all-purpose flour
½ cup (1 stick) margarine at room temperature

10 1-gram packets Equal or Sweet One sugar substitute
½ teaspoon vanilla extract, almond extract, lemon extract, or other flavoring

Combine water, dry milk, and flour in a pan, and stir until smooth. Cook, stirring constantly, over medium heat until mixture is thick and smooth, or cook in a microwave oven for 2 minutes, stirring every 30 seconds. Place the pan in cold water and stir mixture until cool. Set aside.

Cream margarine and sugar substitute together until light and fluffy. Add cooled flour mixture, 1 tablespoon at a time, while beating at medium speed. Add flavoring and beat at high speed until light and fluffy. Refrigerate until used, on cooled cake. Calculate 1 tablespoon per serving (¾ cup for 12 servings; 1 cup for 16 servings). Makes 1¼ cups.

Yield: 20 (1-tablespoon) servings
Food exchanges per serving: 1 fat; or no carbohydrate choices
Sugar per serving: None
Low-cholesterol diets: Recipe is suitable as written.
Low-sodium diets: Use salt-free margarine.
Nutritive values per serving:

Calories: 48
CHO: 1 g
PRO: negligible

FAT: 5 g
Na: 56 mg
Cholesterol: 0

CHAPTER 6

Cookies

WE'VE HAD MANY people tell us they miss their cookie jars more than anything else now that they have diabetes. Most traditional cookies are high in carbohydrates and fat. We resolved some time ago to develop and publish cookie recipes that would fit into a diabetes meal plan; we hope you will like these as much as our friends and family do.

We also decided to include in these recipes everything possible to make really good cookies. We've gone all out; instead of trying to get two cookies for a carbohydrate choice or starch exchange, we've attempted to fit all of the goodies we could into cookies that are each worth a carbohydrate choice or one starch and one fat exchange. The carbohydrate choice accounts for the sugar and flour in the cookies, and a small amount of fat is a necessary trade-off for their texture and flavor.

Because many people with diabetes are concerned with cholesterol, we have added tips explaining how to modify recipes for low-cholesterol and low-sodium diets.

The same basic principles for good baking that apply to cookies with higher fat and sugar content apply to these cookies. Here are some that you should remember:

1. Read the recipe before beginning to bake, and make sure you understand it and have all of the ingredients on hand. In fact, it's a good idea to measure the ingredients before you start the actual preparation.
2. Preheat the oven as long as necessary before combining ingredi-

ents, usually about 10 minutes before you begin the mixing. Ovens do vary, so you should regulate yours according to past experience.

3. Follow the recipe exactly when you are preparing carbohydrate-controlled foods. Do not add any other ingredients unless you know how to calculate the additions and establish new nutritive and exchange values.

4. Ingredients should be at room temperature unless the recipe says otherwise. This is especially true for eggs and liquid egg substitute and for margarine, which is much easier to cream if it has been out of the refrigerator for at least 15 to 20 minutes.

5. Flour should not be sifted unless the recipe tells you to do so, since there is a difference in the weight of sifted and unsifted flour. We usually stir the flour and other ingredients together to blend them, which gives you the same results as sifting them and is a lot simpler to do.

6. Cookies should not be overbaked, because they lose their flavor rapidly if they bake too long. Transfer cookies as instructed from cookie sheets to a wire rack to cool, because they will continue to bake if left on the hot cookie sheets.

7. Use standard measuring cups and spoons, and bake cookies at the temperature indicated in the recipe.

8. Cookies (the cookie dough, that is) should be of uniform size, and uniformly placed on a cookie sheet so they will bake evenly. If you don't have enough dough to fill a cookie sheet, put the cookies in the center of the cookie sheet and bake according to the directions in the recipe.

9. Good-quality cookie sheets are essential. Poor-quality sheets will buckle in the oven and cookies won't bake evenly. Cookie sheets with a nonstick surface make cookie baking much easier; the surface is easier to spray or grease, and to clean. I like to use a cooking spray on cookie sheets; it's simpler and less messy and it means less fat in your cookies.

10. You may sometimes need to press the cookie dough down to a required thickness because the dough doesn't include enough sugar and fat for the cookies to spread while they are baking. Baking powder and baking soda also help cookies rise and spread while they are baking. It is important to have enough liquid in the dough to help other ingredients do their job.

11. Always use ingredients of good quality: you get out of finished cookies exactly what you put into the dough. In addition, take good care of cookies after they are baked. Some freeze well and can be thawed in their container in the refrigerator. Others, such as macaroons, should be stored for a shorter time, loosely covered, at room temperature. If you intend to keep them a long time, you can freeze them.

We mention a no. 60 dipper (1 level tablespoon) and a no. 40 dipper (1½ tablespoons) in many of the cookie recipes. These are like ice cream dippers and can be bought in a hardware or kitchen equipment store (if the store doesn't have them, perhaps it will order them for you). The number on the dipper refers to the number of dipperfuls in a quart, so the larger number (60) means a smaller dipper and the smaller number (40) means a larger dipper. We suggest you use them if you plan to make a lot of cookies; they will give you uniform size.

Almond Biscotti

Slivered almonds and almond extract add a rich flavor to these biscotti.

¾ cup sugar
⅓ cup vegetable oil
2 tablespoons applesauce
1 cup egg whites or liquid
  egg substitute
1 teaspoon almond extract

2 tablespoons water
4½ cups all-purpose flour
1 tablespoon baking
  powder
⅓ cup slivered almonds
2 tablespoons fat-free milk

Using an electric mixer at medium speed, beat sugar, oil, applesauce, egg whites or liquid egg substitute, almond extract, and water until well blended. Stir flour and baking powder together and add to the creamy mixture. Mix at medium speed to blend. Stir in slivered almonds.

Turn dough out onto a floured work surface and knead briefly. Divide dough into two equal portions and form each portion into a roll 15 inches long. Place rolls on cookie sheet that has been sprayed with cooking spray or lined with aluminum foil. Brush with milk.

Bake at 375°F for 15 to 30 minutes, or until lightly browned. Cool 5 minutes on a wire rack. While warm, slice each roll into 20 diagonal slices, each about ¾ inch thick.

Place slices on their sides on ungreased cookie sheets and bake for 5 minutes, turn, and bake for another 5 minutes. Cool on wire racks.

Note: Biscotti may be stored in an airtight container at room temperature or frozen almost indefinitely. They are generally made 2 or 3 days before they are needed, then allowed to stand to develop their flavor.

Yield: 42 cookies
Food exchanges per cookie: 1 starch; or 1 carbohydrate choice
Sugar per cookie: 1 teaspoon or 4 grams
Low-cholesterol diets: Recipe is suitable as written.
Low-sodium diets: Use low-sodium baking powder.
Nutritive values per cookie:

Calories: 80
CHO: 14 g
PRO: 2 g

FAT: 2 g
Na: 45 mg
Cholesterol: 0

Biscotti

These firm, crisp Italian cookies are generally served with wine or coffee. This recipe came from my husband's cousin Mary Cavaiani Lancour, from Iron Mountain, Michigan.

¾ cup sugar
⅓ cup vegetable oil
2 tablespoons unsweetened applesauce
1 cup egg whites or liquid egg substitute

1 teaspoon anise flavoring
4½ cups all-purpose flour
1 tablespoon baking powder
2 tablespoons fat-free milk

Using an electric mixer at medium speed, beat sugar, oil, applesauce, egg whites or liquid egg substitute, and anise flavoring together to blend well. Stir flour and baking powder together and add to the creamy mixture. Mix at medium speed to blend.

Turn dough out onto a floured work surface and knead briefly. Divide dough into two equal portions and form each portion into a roll 15 inches long. Place rolls on cookie sheet that has been sprayed with cooking spray or lined with aluminum foil. Brush with milk.

Bake at 375°F for 25 to 30 minutes, or until firm and lightly browned. Cool 5 minutes on a wire rack. Then, while warm, slice each roll into 20 diagonal slices, each about ¾ inch thick.

Place slices on their sides on ungreased cookie sheets and bake for 5 minutes, turn, and bake for another 5 minutes. Cool on wire racks.

Note: Biscotti may be stored in an airtight container at room temperature or frozen indefinitely. They are generally made 2 or 3 days before they are needed, then allowed to stand to develop their flavor.

Yield: 42 cookies
Food exchanges per cookie: 1 starch; or 1 carbohydrate choice
Sugar per cookie: 1 teaspoon or 4 grams
Low-cholesterol diets: Recipe is suitable as written.
Low-sodium diets: Use low-sodium baking powder.
Nutritive values per cookie:

Calories: 80
CHO: 14 g
PRO: 2 g

FAT: 2 g
Na: 45 mg
Cholesterol: 0

Cardamom Slices

These cookies are exceptionally good with a hot cup of cappuccino on a cold winter day. This recipe makes a very large batch.

1½ cups sugar
¾ cup (1½ sticks) margarine at room temperature
1 teaspoon vanilla extract
2 tablespoons unsweetened applesauce

6 large eggs (1½ cups eggs or egg substitute)
6 cups all-purpose flour
1 tablespoon baking powder
2 teaspoons ground cardamom
¼ cup chopped nuts (optional)

In a mixing bowl, cream sugar, margarine, and vanilla. Add applesauce and mix well. Add eggs, 2 at a time, beating well after each addition.

Stir flour, baking powder, and cardamom together to blend. Add to creamed mixture. Add nuts if using and mix lightly. Roll the dough into 4 12-inch-long rolls. Place rolls on cookie sheet that has been sprayed with cooking spray or lined with aluminum foil. Brush with milk.

Bake at 350°F for 20 to 25 minutes, or until firm enough to cut.

While warm, cut diagonally into ½-inch slices, lay cookies on their sides on ungreased cookie sheets, and bake an additional 5 to 10 minutes at 250°F until very lightly browned.

Yield: 96 cookies
Food exchanges per cookie: ½ starch; or ½ carbohydrate choice
Sugar per cookie: .75 teaspoon or 3 grams
Low-cholesterol diets: Omit eggs. Use liquid egg substitute.
Low-sodium diets: Use low-sodium baking powder.
Nutritive values per cookie:

Calories: 65	FAT: 3 g
CHO: 9 g	Na: 40 mg
PRO: 2 g	Cholesterol: 15 mg

Chocolate Coconut Macaroons

I don't use a dipper for these cookies; I get better results when I drop them from a spoon. This recipe is a little different from most macaroons, but they are very good and they are very easy to make.

¼ cup semisweet chocolate chips
2 large egg whites
¼ teaspoon cream of tartar
½ cup sugar
1 teaspoon vanilla extract

1 teaspoon chocolate flavoring (optional)
⅛ teaspoon salt
2⅓ cups sweetened, flaked coconut

Melt chocolate chips in the top of a double boiler or in a microwave oven. Set aside and cool to room temperature.

Place egg whites and cream of tartar in a mixer bowl and beat at high speed, using a whip, until peaks are formed. Add sugar gradually while continuing to beat at high speed. Add flavorings and salt to meringue, beating at slow speed. Add melted chocolate, continuing to beat at slow speed. Remove the whip and stir the coconut into the meringue with a spoon. Drop by heaping tablespoonfuls onto cookie sheets that have been sprayed with cooking spray or lined with aluminum foil.

Bake at 325°F for about 20 minutes, or until macaroons are not quite firm. Remove macaroons to a wire rack and cool to room temperature. Keep in a loosely covered container in a dry place at room temperature, or freeze until needed. Do not cover tightly if storing at room temperature.

Yield: 20 cookies
Food exchanges per cookie: ⅔ starch and 1 fat; or 1 carbohydrate choice
Sugar per cookie: 1.2 teaspoons or 5 grams
Low-cholesterol diets: Use your discretion in deciding to include it in your diet.
Low-sodium diets: Omit salt.
Nutritive values per cookie:

Calories: 86
CHO: 10 g
PRO: 1 g

FAT: 5 g
Na: 22 mg
Cholesterol: 0

Chocolate–Peanut Butter Dreams

The cookies are so chocolately delicious that no one ever guesses they are lower in sugar.

1¼ cups packed brown sugar
1 cup peanut butter, preferably chunky
⅔ cup (1⅓ sticks) margarine at room temperature
⅓ cup water
2 tablespoons unsweetened applesauce

1 large egg
1 teaspoon vanilla extract
3 cups rolled oats
1½ cups all-purpose flour
½ teaspoon baking soda
Sugar

Topping

1½ cups semisweet chocolate chips
4 tablespoons vegetable shortening

⅓ cup chopped nuts (optional)

Beat together brown sugar, peanut butter, and margarine until light and fluffy. Blend in water, applesauce, egg, and vanilla. Combine oats, flour, and soda, add to brown sugar mixture, and mix well. Shape dough into 1-inch balls. Place on ungreased cookie sheets; flatten to ¼-inch thickness with bottom of glass dipped in sugar.

Bake at 350°F for 8 to 10 minutes, or until edges are golden brown. Cool completely.

For topping: In heavy saucepan, over low heat, melt chocolate and vegetable shortening; stir until mixture is melted and smooth. Top each cookie with ½ teaspoon melted chocolate; sprinkle with chopped nuts if using. Chill until set. Store in airtight container.

Yield: 72 cookies
Food exchanges per cookie: 1 starch and ½ fat; or 1 carbohydrate choice
Sugar per cookie: 1.7 teaspoons or 7 grams
Low-cholesterol diets: Omit egg. Use ¼ cup egg whites or liquid egg substitute.
Low-sodium diets: Use salt-free margarine. If possible may also want to use low-sodium peanut butter.
Nutritive values per cookie:

Calories: 105
CHO: 12 g
PRO: 2 g

FAT: 6 g
Na: 50 mg
Cholesterol: 5 mg

Coconut Macaroons

My husband, Chuck, was very fond of the original version of these cookies. We used to buy them in Italian stores before I developed diabetes and needed to make my own. He said mine were very good also!

½ cup all-purpose flour
2 cups sweetened, flaked coconut
½ cup egg whites at room temperature

½ teaspoon cream of tartar
1 cup powdered sugar
1 teaspoon coconut flavoring

Stir flour and coconut together and set aside for later use.

Whip egg whites and cream of tartar together at high speed until stiff peaks form. Add powdered sugar gradually while continuing to whip at medium speed; then add flavoring at low speed. Remove the whip and, with the paddle, carefully add flour mixture at low speed.

Drop mixture by 1½ tablespoonfuls (level no. 40 dipper) onto cookie sheets that have been sprayed with cooking spray or greased with margarine and lightly floured.

Bake at 325°F for about 25 minutes, or until macaroons are firm and lightly browned. Remove macaroons to a wire rack and cool to room temperature. Keep in a loosely covered container at room temperature, or freeze until needed. Do not cover tightly if storing at room temperature.

Yield: 20 cookies
Food exchanges per cookie: ⅔ starch and ½ fat; or 1 carbohydrate choice
Sugar per cookie: 1.2 teaspoons or 5 grams
Low-cholesterol diets: Use only 1 cup coconut. Use your discretion in deciding to include it in your diet.
Low-sodium diets: Recipe is suitable as written.
Nutritive values per cookie:

Calories: 62	FAT: 3 g
CHO: 9 g	Na: 12 mg
PRO: 1 g	Cholesterol: 0

Krispie Almond Meringues

These cookies should be stored, if you have any left to store, loosely covered in a dry place.

½ cup egg whites at room
   temperature
¼ teaspoon cream of tartar
1 cup sugar

1½ teaspoons almond
   extract
3 cups Kellogg's Rice Krispies
1 cup chopped almonds

Place egg whites and cream of tartar in a mixer bowl and beat at high speed, using a whip, until peaks are formed. Add sugar slowly, while continuing to beat at high speed. Blend flavoring into meringue. Remove the whip and add Rice Krispies and almonds, using a spoon to stir them together. Drop dough by 1½ tablespoonfuls (level no. 40 dipper) onto cookie sheets that have been sprayed with cooking spray or lined with aluminum foil. Press meringues down lightly with the back of a tablespoon dipped in cold water.

Bake at 325°F for about 25 minutes, or until meringues are lightly browned and firm. Remove meringues to a wire rack and cool to room temperature.

Yield: 48 cookies
Food exchanges per cookie: ½ starch; or ½ carbohydrate choice
Sugar per cookie: 1 teaspoon or 4 grams
Low-cholesterol diets: Recipe is suitable as written.
Low-sodium diets: Recipe is suitable as written.
Nutritive values per cookie:

Calories: 40
CHO: 6 g
PRO: 1 g

FAT: 2 g
Na: 22 mg
Cholesterol: 0

Pecan Dainties

This recipe is from Florence Jellings, of Arlington, Iowa, who once brought the cookies along to a tea party. I was thrilled to discover they fit into a carbohydrate-controlled diet. They aren't really big, but they have a wonderful texture and flavor.

2 large egg whites
¼ teaspoon cream of tartar
1 cup packed brown sugar

1 teaspoon vanilla extract
1 cup chopped pecans
1½ cups cornflakes

Beat egg whites and cream of tartar at high speed with a whip, until stiff. Add brown sugar gradually, while continuing to beat at high speed, to form a meringue. Add vanilla at slow speed. Remove the whip and add pecans and cornflakes with a large spoon or spatula. Drop by 1½ tablespoonfuls (level no. 40 dipper) onto cookie sheets that have been sprayed with cooking spray or lined with aluminum foil.

Bake at 250°F for about 30 minutes, or until firm. Remove to a wire rack and cool to room temperature. Store in a loosely covered container at room temperature, or freeze until needed. Do not store in a tightly covered container at room temperature, or they will become soft.

Yield: 24 cookies
Food exchanges per cookie: 1 starch and ½ fat; or 1 carbohydrate choice
Sugar per cookie: 2 teaspoons or 8 grams
Low-cholesterol diets: Recipe is suitable as written.
Low-sodium diets: Recipe is suitable as written.
Nutritive values per cookie:

Calories: 86
CHO: 14 g
PRO: 1 g

FAT: 3 g
Na: 74 mg
Cholesterol: 0

Chipless Cookies

These are great—they taste like chocolate chip cookies without the chocolate chips.

2/3 cup (1 1/3 sticks) margarine at room temperature
2/3 cup sugar
1/3 cup liquid egg substitute
1 tablespoon unsweetened applesauce

1 1/2 teaspoons vanilla extract
2 1/2 cups all-purpose flour
1 teaspoon baking powder
1 teaspoon salt
1/4 cup chopped pecans
1/4 cup raisins

Using an electric mixer at medium speed, cream margarine and sugar together until light and fluffy. Add liquid egg substitute and vanilla and mix at medium speed for 30 seconds, scraping down the bowl before and after the addition.

Stir flour, baking powder, salt, pecans, and raisins together and add to the creamy mixture. Mix at medium speed to blend. Drop dough by 1 1/2 tablespoonfuls (level no. 40 dipper) onto baking sheets that have been sprayed with cooking spray or lined with foil, and flatten slightly.

Bake at 375°F for 10 minutes, or until lightly browned. Cool on wire racks.

Yield: 36 cookies
Food exchanges per cookie: 1 starch; or 1 carbohydrate choice
Sugar per cookie: 1 teaspoon or 4 grams
Low-cholesterol diets: Recipe is suitable as written.
Low-sodium diets: Omit salt. Use low-sodium baking powder.
Nutritive values per cookie:

Calories: 90
CHO: 15 g
PRO: 1 g

FAT: 4 g
Na: 120 mg
Cholesterol: 0

Anna's Chocolate Chip Cookies

Like most little girls, Anna Daab loves chocolate chip cookies, so her mother, Diane, developed this recipe for her, using vegetable oil instead of margarine.

2 cups all-purpose flour
½ cup granulated sugar
½ cup packed brown sugar
1 teaspoon baking soda
½ cup vegetable oil

⅓ cup egg whites
1 teaspoon vanilla extract
2 tablespoons water
1 cup semisweet chocolate chips

Place flour, sugars, and baking soda in a mixer bowl and mix at low speed to blend well. Add oil, egg whites, vanilla, water, and chocolate chips, and mix at medium speed to blend. Drop dough by tablespoonfuls (level no. 60 dipper) onto cookie sheets that have been sprayed with cooking spray or lined with aluminum foil.

Bake at 375°F for about 10 minutes, or until cookies are lightly browned. Remove them to a wire rack and cool to room temperature.

Yield: 30 cookies
Food exchanges per cookie: 1 starch and 1 fat; or 1 carbohydrate choice
Sugar per cookie: 1.6 teaspoons or 7 grams
Low-cholesterol diets: Recipe is suitable as written.
Low-sodium diets: Recipe is suitable as written.
Nutritive values per cookie:

Calories: 119
CHO: 16 g
PRO: 1 g

FAT: 6 g
Na: 35 mg
Cholesterol: 0

Chocolate Chip Cookies

I can't imagine an American cookbook without a chocolate chip cookie recipe. These cost a starch and a fat exchange or one carbohydrate choice, but I think they are worth it.

½ cup (1 stick) margarine at room temperature
⅓ cup packed brown sugar
⅓ cup granulated sugar
1 teaspoon vanilla extract
1 large egg

1¼ cups all-purpose flour
¼ teaspoon baking soda
¼ teaspoon salt
½ cup chopped English walnuts
½ cup semisweet chocolate chips

Cream margarine and sugars together at medium speed until light and fluffy. Add vanilla and egg, and mix at medium speed for 1 minute, scraping down the bowl before and after adding them. Stir flour, baking soda, salt, walnuts, and chocolate chips together; add to creamy mixture. Mix at medium speed for about 30 seconds, or until blended. Drop dough by 1½ tablespoonfuls (level no. 40 dipper) onto cookie sheets that have been sprayed with cooking spray or lined with aluminum foil.

Bake at 375°F for 10 to 12 minutes, or until cookies are lightly browned. Leave them on sheets for 3 minutes; then remove cookies to a wire rack and cool to room temperature.

Yield: 20 cookies
Food exchanges per cookie: 1 starch and 1 fat; or 1 carbohydrate choice
Sugar per cookie: 1.6 teaspoons or 7 grams
Low-cholesterol diets: Omit egg. Use ¼ cup egg whites or liquid egg substitute.
Low-sodium diets: Omit salt. Use salt-free margarine.
Nutritive values per cookie:

Calories: 109
CHO: 11 g
PRO: 1 g

FAT: 7 g
Na: 127 mg
Cholesterol: 13 mg

Lemon Chocolate Chip Cookies

I like this taste combination, with its contrast of chocolate and lemon flavors.

1/4 cup sugar
1/2 cup dry lemonade mix (not sugar-free)
1/2 cup (1 stick) margarine at room temperature
2 tablespoons light corn syrup
1 large egg

1/4 cup water at room temperature
2 1/2 cups all-purpose flour
1/2 teaspoon baking powder
1/4 teaspoon baking soda
1/4 teaspoon salt
1/2 cup semisweet chocolate chips

Mix sugar, lemonade mix, margarine, and corn syrup together at medium speed until creamy. Add egg and water, and mix at medium speed for 30 seconds, scraping down the bowl before and after adding them. Stir flour, baking powder, baking soda, salt, and chocolate chips together to blend. Add to sugar mixture and mix at medium speed until creamy. Drop dough by 1 1/2 tablespoonfuls (level no. 40 dipper) onto cookie sheets that have been sprayed with cooking spray or lined with aluminum foil. Press each cookie down to 1/3-inch thickness with the back of a tablespoon dipped in cold water.

Bake at 350°F for about 12 to 14 minutes, or until cookies are lightly browned on the bottom. Remove to a wire rack and cool to room temperature.

Yield: 30 cookies
Food exchanges per cookie: 1 starch and 1 fat; or 1 carbohydrate choice
Sugar per cookie: 1.4 teaspoons or 6 grams
Low-cholesterol diets: Omit egg. Use 1/4 cup egg whites or liquid egg substitute.
Low-sodium diets: Omit salt. Use salt-free margarine and low-sodium baking powder.
Nutritive values per cookie:

Calories: 113
CHO: 17 g
PRO: 2 g

FAT: 5 g
Na: 75 mg
Cholesterol: 10 mg

Orange Chocolate Chip Cookies

This recipe is based on one from my friend Mary Boineau, of Tampa, Florida. She loves to bake cakes and cookies for her family, friends, and bowling group, and her idea of a perfect gift is a cake or cookie cookbook.

¼ cup (½ stick) margarine at
    room temperature
¼ cup sugar
¼ cup dry orange-flavored
    breakfast drink mix (not
    sugar-free)
Dry sugar substitute equal to ⅓
    cup sugar
1 large egg

1 teaspoon orange flavoring
1½ cups all-purpose flour
¼ cup instant nonfat dry milk
½ teaspoon baking soda
½ teaspoon salt
1 cup semisweet chocolate
    chips
½ cup water at room
    temperature

Cream margarine, sugar, drink mix, and dry sugar substitute together at medium speed until light and fluffy. Add egg and flavoring, and mix at medium speed until creamy. Stir flour, dry milk, baking soda, and salt together to blend; add, along with chocolate chips and water, to creamy mixture. Mix at medium speed until well blended. Drop dough by 1½ tablespoonfuls (level no. 40 dipper) onto cookie sheets that have been sprayed with cooking spray or lined with aluminum foil.

Bake at 375°F for 12 to 15 minutes, or until cookies are firm, and lightly browned on the bottom. Remove them to a wire rack and cool to room temperature.

Yield: 24 cookies
Food exchanges per cookie: 1 starch and 1 fat; or 1 carbohydrate
    choice
Sugar per cookie: 1.6 teaspoons or 7 grams
Low-cholesterol diets: Omit egg. Use ¼ cup egg whites or liquid egg
    substitute.
Low-sodium diets: Omit salt. Use salt-free margarine.
Nutritive values per cookie:

Calories: 108	FAT: 5 g
CHO: 15 g	Na: 99 mg
PRO: 2 g	Cholesterol: 11 mg

Pecan Chocolate Chip Cookies

Black walnuts, which grow profusely in our area, are also good in these cookies. You can substitute them for the pecans with no effect on the nutritive or exchange values.

½ cup (1 stick) margarine at room temperature
1 cup packed brown sugar
¼ cup egg whites
1 teaspoon vanilla extract
2 tablespoons water
2 cups all-purpose flour

1 tablespoon instant nonfat dry milk
½ teaspoon salt
¾ teaspoon baking soda
½ cup semisweet chocolate chips
⅓ cup chopped pecans

Cream margarine and brown sugar together at medium speed until light and fluffy. Add egg whites, vanilla, and water, and mix at medium speed for 1 minute, scraping down the bowl before and after adding them. Stir flour, dry milk, salt, and baking soda together to blend well; add, along with chocolate chips and pecans, to creamed mixture. Mix at medium speed to blend. Drop dough by 1½ tablespoonfuls (level no. 40 dipper) onto cookie sheets that have been sprayed with cooking spray or lined with aluminum foil.

Bake at 375°F for 10 to 12 minutes, or until cookies are lightly browned. Leave them on the cookie sheets for 2 minutes; then remove cookies to a wire rack and cool to room temperature.

Yield: 30 cookies
Food exchanges per cookie: 1 starch and 1 fat; or 1 carbohydrate choice
Sugar per cookie: 1.6 teaspoons or 7 grams
Low-cholesterol diets: Recipe is suitable as written.
Low-sodium diets: Omit salt. Use salt-free margarine.
Nutritive values per cookie:

Calories: 108
CHO: 15 g
PRO: 1 g

FAT: 5 g
Na: 100 mg
Cholesterol: 0

Peanut Butter Chocolate Chip Cookies

Chocolate and peanut butter are two favorite flavors that go together well in candy, once in a while in a pie—and in these tasty treats.

1/4 cup (1/2 stick) margarine at room temperature
3/4 cup sugar
1/2 cup chunky peanut butter
Dry sugar substitute equal to 1/4 cup sugar (optional)
1/3 cup egg whites

1 teaspoon vanilla extract
1/4 cup water
1 1/2 cups all-purpose flour
3/4 teaspoon baking soda
1/2 teaspoon salt
1/2 cup semisweet chocolate chips

Cream margarine, sugar, peanut butter, and dry sugar substitute (if using) together at medium speed until light and fluffy. Add egg whites, vanilla, and water, and mix at medium speed for 30 seconds, scraping down the bowl before and after adding these ingredients. Stir flour, baking soda, salt, and chocolate chips together to blend well (don't break up the chips). Add to creamy mixture, and mix to blend. Drop dough by 1 1/2 tablespoonfuls (level no. 40 dipper) onto cookie sheets that have been sprayed with cooking spray or lined with aluminum foil.

Bake at 350°F for 10 to 12 minutes, or until cookies are lightly browned. Leave them on sheets for 3 to 4 minutes; then remove cookies to a wire rack and cool to room temperature.

Yield: 24 cookies
Food exchanges per cookie: 1 starch and 1 fat; or 1 carbohydrate choice
Sugar per cookie: 1.5 teaspoons or 6 grams
Low-cholesterol diets: Recipe is suitable as written.
Low-sodium diets: Omit salt. Use salt-free margarine and low-sodium peanut butter, if possible.
Nutritive values per cookie:

Calories: 121	FAT: 6 g
CHO: 15 g	Na: 124 mg
PRO: 3 g	Cholesterol: 0

Whole-Wheat Chocolate Chip Cookies

This recipe is based on cookies prepared by the dietary department at the Lutheran Nursing Home in Strawberry Point, Iowa. I was the nutrition consultant there for several years, and we always tried to get as much fiber into the residents' diets as possible, frequently using whole-wheat flour. These cookies have a rich buttery taste, and the residents enjoyed them for dessert or with their afternoon coffee.

³/₄ cup whole-wheat flour
³/₄ cup all-purpose flour
¹/₂ cup packed brown sugar
¹/₂ teaspoon baking soda
¹/₂ teaspoon baking powder
¹/₂ teaspoon salt
¹/₂ teaspoon cinnamon

Dry sugar substitute equal to ¹/₃ cup sugar
¹/₃ cup vegetable oil
1 large egg
1 tablespoon molasses
¹/₄ cup water
³/₄ cup semisweet chocolate chips
¹/₂ cup raisins

Place flours, brown sugar, baking soda, baking powder, salt, cinnamon, and dry sugar substitute in a mixer bowl and mix at low speed to blend well. Beat oil, egg, molasses, and water together with a fork to blend; and then add, along with chocolate chips and raisins, to flour mixture. Mix until all flour is moistened. Drop dough by tablespoonfuls (level no. 60 dipper) onto cookie sheets that have been sprayed with cooking spray or lined with aluminum foil.

Bake at 350°F for 12 to 15 minutes, or until cookies are firm. Leave cookies on cookie sheets for 1 to 2 minutes; then remove cookies to a wire rack and cool to room temperature.

Yield: 28 cookies
Food exchanges per cookie: 1 starch and 1 fat; or 1 carbohydrate choice
Sugar per cookie: .9 teaspoon or 4 grams
Low-cholesterol diets: Omit egg. Use ¹/₄ cup egg whites or liquid egg substitute.
Low-sodium diets: Omit salt. Use low-sodium baking powder.
Nutritive values per cookie:

Calories: 95
CHO: 14 g
PRO: 1 g
FAT: 5 g
Na: 65 mg
Cholesterol: 10 mg

Anna's Cereal Cookies

Anna Daab's mother, Diane, who gave me this recipe, sometimes substitutes other cereals that have the same amount of carbohydrate per cup as the cornflakes and Rice Krispies.

1 cup rolled oats
3/4 cup cornflakes
3/4 cup Kellogg's Rice
    Krispies
1 cup packed brown sugar
3/4 cup vegetable oil

1/4 cup egg whites
1 teaspoon vanilla extract
2 1/2 cups all-purpose flour
1 teaspoon baking soda
1 tablespoon instant nonfat dry
    milk

Combine oats and cereals, and mix lightly. Set aside for later use.

Place brown sugar, oil, egg whites, and vanilla in a mixer bowl and mix at medium speed to blend well. Stir flour, baking soda, and dry milk together to blend; add to creamy mixture. Mix at medium speed to blend; add cereal mixture. Mix only until cereal is absorbed into the dough. Drop dough by tablespoonfuls (level no. 60 dipper) onto cookie sheets that have been sprayed with cooking spray or lined with aluminum foil. Press each cookie down to 1/2-inch thickness with the back of a tablespoon dipped in cold water.

Bake at 350°F for 10 to 12 minutes, or until cookies are browned and firm. Remove them to a wire rack and cool to room temperature.

Yield: 36 cookies
Food exchanges per cookie: 1 starch; or 1 carbohydrate choice
Sugar per cookie: 1.3 teaspoons or 5 grams
Low-cholesterol diets: Recipe is suitable as written.
Low-sodium diets: Recipe is suitable as written.
Nutritive values per cookie:

Calories: 87
CHO: 16 g
PRO: 2 g

FAT: 2 g
Na: 58 mg
Cholesterol: 0

Cereal Cookies

I have always liked these cookies, and I enjoy them even more since I started using almond extract instead of vanilla.

½ cup granulated sugar
½ cup packed brown
   sugar
1 cup (2 sticks) margarine at
   room temperature
1 teaspoon almond extract
⅓ cup egg whites

2 cups all-purpose flour
1 teaspoon baking powder
1 teaspoon baking soda
2 cups rolled oats
½ cup raisins
½ cup All-Bran, Bran Buds,
   Fiber One, or 100% Bran

Cream sugars and margarine together at medium speed until light and fluffy. Add flavoring and egg whites, and mix at medium speed until creamy, scraping down the bowl before and after addition. Stir flour, baking powder, and baking soda together to blend well; add to creamy mixture. Mix at medium speed until flour is absorbed; add oats, raisins, and cereal, and mix to blend. Drop dough by 1½ tablespoonfuls (level no. 40 dipper) onto cookie sheets that have been sprayed with cooking spray or lined with aluminum foil. Press each cookie down to ½-inch thickness with the back of a tablespoon dipped in cold water.

Bake at 350°F for 10 to 12 minutes, or until cookies are lightly browned. Remove them to a wire rack and cool to room temperature.

Yield: 36 cookies
Food exchanges per cookie: 1 starch and 1 fat; or 1 carbohydrate
   choice
Sugar per cookie: 1.3 teaspoons or 5 grams
Low-cholesterol diets: Recipe is suitable as written.
Low-sodium diets: Omit salt. Use salt-free margarine and low-sodium
   baking powder.
Nutritive values per cookie:

Calories: 119   FAT: 5 g
CHO: 16 g   Na: 106 mg
PRO: 2 g   Cholesterol: 0

Chocolate Oatmeal Cookies

This luscious chocolate cookie also has fiber in it, thanks to the oatmeal.

1 cup granulated sugar
1 cup packed brown sugar
3/4 cup (1 1/2 sticks) margarine at room temperature
2 large eggs
2 teaspoons vanilla extract
2 cups all-purpose flour

1/4 cup unsweetened cocoa powder
1 teaspoon baking soda
1/2 teaspoon baking powder
1/2 teaspoon salt
1/4 cup water
2 cups rolled oats

Cream sugars and margarine together at medium speed until light and fluffy. Add eggs and vanilla, and beat at medium speed until creamy again, scraping down the bowl before and after addition. Stir flour, cocoa, baking soda, baking powder, and salt together to blend well. Add to creamy mixture; mix at medium speed only until flour is moistened. Add water and oats, and mix at medium speed until oats are absorbed into the dough. Drop dough by tablespoonfuls (level no. 60 dipper) onto cookie sheets that have been sprayed with cooking spray or lined with aluminum foil.

Bake at 375°F for 10 to 12 minutes, or until cookies are almost firm in the center. Leave them on sheets for 3 to 4 minutes; then remove cookies to a wire rack and cool to room temperature.

Yield: 48 cookies
Food exchanges per cookie: 1 starch and 1/2 fat; or 1 carbohydrate choice
Sugar per cookie: 2 teaspoons or 8 grams
Low-cholesterol diets: Omit eggs. Use 1/2 cup egg whites or liquid egg substitute.
Low-sodium diets: Omit salt. Use salt-free margarine and low-sodium baking powder.
Nutritive values per cookie:

Calories: 94
CHO: 15 g
PRO: 1 g

FAT: 3 g
Na: 81 mg
Cholesterol: 11 mg

Double-Chocolate Oatmeal Cookies

This recipe is based on one from my friend Frances Nielsen, of Oak Lawn, Illinois. Frances is a wonderful cook and has taught me so much about cooking.

1 cup sugar
1 cup (2 sticks) margarine at room temperature
1 large egg
¼ cup water
1 teaspoon vanilla extract
1¼ cups all-purpose flour

½ cup whole-wheat flour
¼ cup unsweetened cocoa powder
2 cups rolled oats
½ teaspoon baking soda
½ teaspoon baking powder
½ cup semisweet chocolate chips

Cream sugar and margarine together at medium speed until light and fluffy. Add egg, water, and vanilla, and mix at medium speed for 30 seconds, scraping down the bowl before and after addition. Stir flours, cocoa, oats, baking soda, and baking powder together to blend; add to egg mixture. Mix at medium speed to blend and then add chocolate chips. Drop dough by 1½ tablespoonfuls (level no. 40 dipper) onto cookie sheets that have been sprayed with cooking spray or lined with aluminum foil.

Bake at 350°F for 12 to 14 minutes, or until cookies are not quite firm; *do not overbake,* or cookies will be too hard. Remove them to a wire rack and cool to room temperature.

Yield: 36 cookies
Food exchanges per cookie: 1 starch and 1 fat; or 1 carbohydrate choice
Sugar per cookie: 1.3 teaspoons or 5 grams
Low-cholesterol diets: Omit egg. Use ¼ cup egg whites or liquid egg substitute.
Low-sodium diets: Use salt-free margarine and low-sodium baking powder.
Nutritive values per cookie:

Calories: 120
CHO: 15 g
PRO: 2 g

FAT: 6 g
Na: 77 mg
Cholesterol: 8 mg

Coconut Oatmeal Cookies

1 cup packed brown sugar
¾ cup (1½ sticks) margarine at
  room temperature
2 large eggs
1 teaspoon vanilla extract
1 teaspoon coconut
  flavoring
2 cups all-purpose flour

1½ cups rolled oats
1½ cups sweetened, flaked
  coconut
1 teaspoon baking soda
½ teaspoon baking powder
¼ teaspoon salt
Dry sugar substitute equal to
  ¼ cup sugar

Cream brown sugar and margarine together until light and fluffy. Add eggs and flavorings, and beat at medium speed until creamy, scraping the bowl before and after addition. Stir flour, oats, coconut, baking soda, baking powder, salt, and dry sugar substitute together to blend, and add to creamy mixture. Mix at medium speed until blended. Drop dough by 1½ tablespoonfuls (level no. 40 dipper) onto cookie sheets that have been sprayed with cooking spray or lined with aluminum foil. Press each cookie down lightly with the back of a tablespoon dipped in water.

Bake at 350°F for 12 to 14 minutes, or until cookies are lightly browned. Remove them to a wire rack and cool to room temperature.

Yield: 36 cookies
Food exchanges per cookie: 1 starch and 1 fat; or 1 carbohydrate
  choice
Sugar per cookie: 1.3 teaspoons or 5 grams
Low-cholesterol diets: Use only ¾ cup coconut. Use your discretion in
  deciding to include it in your diet.
Low-sodium diets: Omit salt. Use salt-free margarine and low-sodium
  baking powder.
Nutritive values per cookie:

Calories: 119	FAT: 6 g
CHO: 15 g	Na: 103 mg
PRO: 2 g	Cholesterol: 15 mg

Etta's Oatmeal Cookies

These cookies are a favorite of our cousins Dave and Etta Cavaiani of Iron Mountain, Michigan. Etta brought them along once when we met for a weekend in Wisconsin, and we enjoyed them while we visited.

½ cup (1 stick) margarine at
   room temperature
¼ cup granulated sugar
¼ cup packed brown sugar
Dry sugar substitute equal to ¼
   cup sugar
¼ cup egg whites
1 teaspoon vanilla extract
½ teaspoon black walnut
   flavoring

¼ cup water at room
   temperature
1½ cups all-purpose flour
1 teaspoon baking powder
1 teaspoon baking soda
¼ teaspoon salt
2 cups rolled oats
½ cup chopped black or
   English walnuts
   (optional)

Cream margarine, sugars, and dry sugar substitute together at medium speed until light and fluffy. Add egg whites, flavorings, and water, and mix at medium speed for 30 seconds, scraping down the bowl before and after addition. Stir flour, baking powder, baking soda, salt, oats, and walnuts (if using) together to blend, and add to creamy mixture. Mix to blend. Drop dough by 1½ tablespoonfuls (level no. 40 dipper) onto cookie sheets that have been sprayed with cooking spray or lined with aluminum foil. Press each cookie down lightly with the back of a tablespoon dipped in cold water.

Bake at 350°F for 12 to 14 minutes, or until cookies are lightly browned. Remove them to a wire rack and cool to room temperature.

Yield: 24 cookies
Food exchanges per cookie: 1 starch and 1 fat; or 1 carbohydrate
   choice
Sugar per cookie: 1 teaspoon or 4 grams
Low-cholesterol diets: Recipe is suitable as written.
Low-sodium diets: Omit salt. Use salt-free margarine and low-sodium
   baking powder.
Nutritive values per cookie:

Calories: 122   FAT: 6 g
CHO: 15 g   Na: 120 mg
PRO: 3 g   Cholesterol: 0

Lemon-Oatmeal Crispies

This is another recipe developed by Diane Daab, of Holland, Michigan. The cookies are enjoyed by husband Kerry, sons Zach and Luke, and daughter Anna, who also has diabetes.

⅔ cup vegetable oil
⅔ cup packed brown sugar
½ cup egg whites
2 tablespoons lemon juice
2 tablespoons grated fresh or finely chopped dried lemon rind

1 teaspoon lemon flavoring
1 cup all-purpose flour
1 cup rolled oats
½ teaspoon baking powder
½ teaspoon baking soda
1½ cups Kellogg's Rice Krispies

Place oil and brown sugar in a mixer bowl and mix at medium speed until creamy. Add egg whites, lemon juice, lemon rind, and flavoring, and mix at medium speed to blend well. Stir flour, oats, baking powder, and baking soda together to blend well; add to creamy mixture while beating at medium speed. Stir in cereal. Drop dough by tablespoonfuls (level no. 60 dipper) onto cookie sheets left ungreased or lined with aluminum foil.

Bake at 350°F for 8 to 10 minutes, or until cookies are lightly browned. Remove them to a wire rack and cool to room temperature.

Yield: 36 cookies
Food exchanges per cookie: ⅔ starch and 1 fat; or 1 carbohydrate choice
Sugar per cookie: 0.9 teaspoon or 4 grams
Low-cholesterol diets: Recipe is suitable as written.
Low-sodium diets: Use low-sodium baking powder.
Nutritive values per cookie:

Calories: 87
CHO: 11 g
PRO: 1 g

FAT: 4 g
Na: 66 mg
Cholesterol: 0

Nut and Cereal Cookies

You can cut the ingredient amounts for these cookies in half very easily. I always make a full batch, though, because they are so popular with my family and friends.

1 cup oat bran cereal
1 cup Fiber One
1 cup Bran Flakes
1 cup rolled oats
1 cup raisins
1 cup chopped walnuts
1 cup packed brown sugar
1 cup (2 sticks) margarine at room temperature

2 teaspoons vanilla extract
2 large eggs
2 cups all-purpose flour
1 teaspoon baking powder
1 teaspoon baking soda
½ teaspoon salt
½ cup water at room temperature

Combine cereals, oats, raisins, and walnuts in a bowl; mix lightly. Set aside.

Cream brown sugar and margarine together at medium speed until light and fluffy. Add vanilla and eggs, and mix at medium speed for 1 minute, scraping down the bowl before and after addition. Stir flour, baking powder, baking soda, and salt together to blend well, and add, along with water, to creamy mixture. Mix only to blend; then add the reserved cereal mixture. Mix at medium speed until blended. Drop dough by 1½ tablespoonfuls (level no. 40 dipper) onto cookie sheets that have been sprayed with cooking spray or lined with aluminum foil.

Bake at 375°F for 12 to 14 minutes, or until cookies are lightly browned. Remove to a wire rack and cool to room temperature.

Yield: 48 cookies

Food exchanges per cookie: 1 starch and 1 fat; or 1 carbohydrate choice

Sugar per cookie: 1 teaspoon or 4 grams

Low-cholesterol diets: Omit eggs. Use ½ cup egg whites or liquid egg substitute.

Low-sodium diets: Omit salt. Use salt-free margarine and low-sodium baking powder.

Nutritive values per cookie:

Calories: 121
CHO: 15 g
PRO: 2 g

FAT: 4 g
Na: 90 mg
Cholesterol: 10 mg

Orange Oatmeal Cookies

½ cup (1 stick) margarine at room temperature
⅔ cup sugar
¼ cup dry orange-flavored breakfast drink mix (not sugar-free)
Dry sugar substitute equal to ¼ cup sugar (optional)

1 teaspoon orange flavoring
¼ cup egg whites
1¾ cups all-purpose flour
½ teaspoon baking soda
½ teaspoon salt
2 cups rolled oats

Cream margarine, sugar, drink mix, and dry sugar substitute (if using) together at medium speed until light and fluffy. Add flavoring and egg whites, and beat at medium speed until creamy, scraping the bowl before and after addition. Stir flour, baking soda, salt, and oats together to blend; add to creamy mixture. Mix at medium speed to blend. Drop dough by 1½ tablespoonfuls (level no. 40 dipper) onto cookie sheets that have been sprayed with cooking spray or lined with aluminum foil.

Bake at 350°F for 12 to 14 minutes, or until cookies are lightly browned. Remove them to a wire rack and cool to room temperature.

Yield: 30 cookies
Food exchanges per cookie: 1 starch and ½ fat; or 1 carbohydrate choice
Sugar per cookie: 1.5 teaspoons or 6 grams
Low-cholesterol diets: Recipe is suitable as written.
Low-sodium diets: Omit salt. Use salt-free margarine.
Nutritive values per cookie:

Calories: 98
CHO: 15 g
PRO: 2 g

FAT: 3 g
Na: 88 mg
Cholesterol: 0

Pecan Oatmeal Cookies

Sometimes I use black walnuts in these cookies, which doesn't change the exchanges but makes them taste more like my mother's cookies.

1 cup rolled oats
½ cup All-Bran, Bran Buds, Fiber One, or 100% Bran
¾ cup chopped pecans
½ cup (1 stick) margarine at room temperature
½ cup granulated sugar
½ cup packed brown sugar

¼ cup egg whites
1 teaspoon vanilla extract
3 tablespoons water
1 cup all-purpose flour
½ teaspoon baking powder
½ teaspoon baking soda
¼ teaspoon salt

Place oats, cereal, and pecans in a bowl and mix lightly. Set aside.

Cream margarine and sugars together at medium speed until light and fluffy. Add egg whites, vanilla, and water, and mix at medium speed for 1 minute, scraping down the bowl before and after addition. Stir flour, baking powder, baking soda, and salt together and add to creamy mixture. Mix at medium speed to blend. Add cereal mixture and mix at medium speed only until cereal is blended into dough. Drop dough by 1½ tablespoonfuls (level no. 40 dipper) onto cookie sheets that have been sprayed with cooking spray or lined with aluminum foil.

Bake at 375°F for about 12 minutes, or until cookies are lightly browned. Leave them on sheets for 2 minutes; then remove cookies to a wire rack and cool to room temperature.

Yield: 24 cookies
Food exchanges per cookie: 1 starch and 1 fat; or 1 carbohydrate choice
Sugar per cookie: 2 teaspoons or 8 grams
Low-cholesterol diets: Recipe is suitable as written.
Low-sodium diets: Omit salt. Use salt-free margarine and low-sodium baking powder.
Nutritive values per cookie:

Calories: 127	FAT: 6 g
CHO: 17 g	Na: 139 mg
PRO: 2 g	Cholesterol: 0

Amish Sugar Cookies

I'm not sure why these are called Amish cookies; I've never seen them for sale in the stores in the Amish settlement near me. Whatever the origin of the name, almost everyone I know in my community makes them, and they are very good. Some cooks add chopped nuts or raisins; if you do that, you need to take into account the exchange values for the added ingredients.

½ cup granulated sugar
⅓ cup powdered sugar
¼ cup (½ stick) margarine
⅓ cup vegetable oil
1 large egg
1 teaspoon vanilla
    extract

1 teaspoon lemon or almond
    extract
2 tablespoons water
2¼ cups all-purpose flour
½ teaspoon baking soda
½ teaspoon cream of tartar
½ teaspoon salt

Place sugars, margarine, and oil in a mixer bowl and mix at medium speed until creamy. Add egg, flavorings, and water, and mix at medium speed for 30 seconds, scraping down the bowl before and after addition. Stir remaining ingredients together to blend well; add to creamy mixture and mix at medium speed to blend. Form dough into 24 balls, using 1 tablespoon (level no. 60 dipper) dough per ball. Place balls on cookie sheets that have been sprayed with cooking spray or lined with aluminum foil. Press balls down evenly to ½-inch thickness with the back of a tablespoon dipped in water.

Bake at 375°F for 12 to 14 minutes, or until cookies are browned on the bottom and lightly browned around the edges. Remove cookies to a wire rack and cool to room temperature.

Yield: 24 cookies
Food exchanges per cookie: 1 starch and 1 fat; or 1 carbohydrate choice
Sugar per cookie: 1.3 teaspoons or 5 grams
Low-cholesterol diets: Omit egg. Use ¼ cup egg whites or liquid egg substitute.
Low-sodium diets: Omit salt. Use salt-free margarine.
Nutritive values per cookie:

Calories: 107   FAT: 5g
CHO: 15 g   Na: 50 mg
PRO: 2 g   Cholesterol: 11 mg

Almond Butter Cookies

3 large eggs
½ cup (1 stick) margarine at room temperature
1½ teaspoons almond extract
2¼ cups all-purpose flour
½ cup packed brown sugar

Dry sugar substitute equal to ¼ cup sugar
1 tablespoon baking powder
½ teaspoon salt
½ cup sliced almonds

Place all but the almonds in a mixer bowl in the order listed, and mix at medium speed to blend. Remove dough to a lightly floured work surface, knead lightly, and form into a roll 12 inches long. Wrap in aluminum foil or plastic, and chill until firm.

Slice chilled dough into 24 slices, each ½ inch thick. Dip top of slices into almonds, and place on cookie sheets that have been sprayed with cooking spray or lined with aluminum foil.

Bake at 375°F for 12 to 14 minutes, or until cookies are browned and firm. Remove them to a wire rack and cool to room temperature.

Yield: 24 cookies
Food exchanges per cookie: 1 starch and 1 fat; or 1 carbohydrate choice
Sugar per cookie: 1 teaspoon or 4 grams
Low-cholesterol diets: Omit eggs. Use ¾ cup egg whites or liquid egg substitute.
Low-sodium diets: Omit salt. Use salt-free margarine and low-sodium baking powder.
Nutritive values per cookie:

Calories: 120　　FAT: 6 g
CHO: 14 g　　Na: 141 mg
PRO: 3 g　　Cholesterol: 34 mg

Vera's Buttermilk Cookies

The recipe for these soft, luscious cookies comes from my friend Vera Wilson. Like me, she has to watch her carbohydrate intake, but we both feel comfortable having these cookies with afternoon coffee in her bright kitchen—one of my favorite places for coffee and a treat.

½ cup (1 stick) margarine at room temperature
⅔ cup sugar
Dry sugar substitute equal to ¼ cup sugar
1 large egg
1 teaspoon vanilla extract

2 cups all-purpose flour
2 tablespoons dry buttermilk
1 teaspoon baking soda
¼ teaspoon salt
⅓ cup water at room temperature

Cream margarine, sugar, and dry sugar substitute together at medium speed until light and fluffy. Add egg and vanilla, and mix at medium speed for 30 seconds, scraping down the bowl before and after addition. Stir flour, dry buttermilk, baking soda, and salt together to blend well. Add flour mixture, along with water, to creamy mixture, and mix at medium speed to blend well. Drop dough by 1½ table-spoonfuls (level no. 40 dipper) onto cookie sheets that have been sprayed with cooking spray or lined with aluminum foil. Press cookies down to ½-inch thickness with the back of a tablespoon dipped in cold water.

Bake at 350°F for 12 to 14 minutes, or until cookies are golden brown on the bottom. Remove them to a wire rack and cool to room temperature.

Yield: 24 cookies
Food exchanges per cookie: 1 starch and 1 fat; or 1 carbohydrate choice
Sugar per cookie: 1.3 teaspoons or 5 grams
Low-cholesterol diets: Omit egg. Use ¼ cup egg whites or liquid egg substitute.
Low-sodium diets: Omit salt. Use salt-free margarine.
Nutritive values per cookie:

Calories: 96   FAT: 4 g
CHO: 13 g   Na: 107 mg
PRO: 2 g   Cholesterol: 12 mg

Chocolate Peppermint Cookies

The nutritive values listed for these cookies are based on using a 2½-inch round cookie cutter. You may use fancy cutters, if you like, as long as each cookie weighs about 1 ounce. You can also add other flavorings such as rum, cherry, and nut flavorings. However, you can't add nuts, raisins, and the like without changing the nutritive values for each cookie.

1 cup (2 sticks) margarine at room temperature
1⅓ cups sugar
1 teaspoon vanilla extract
1 teaspoon peppermint flavoring
½ cup egg whites at room temperature

3 cups all-purpose flour
⅓ cup unsweetened cocoa powder
2 teaspoons baking powder
¼ teaspoon salt

Cream margarine and sugar together at medium speed until light and fluffy. Add flavorings and egg whites, and mix at medium speed for 1 minute, scraping down the bowl before and after addition. Stir flour, cocoa, baking powder, and salt together to blend well; add to creamy mixture. Mix at medium speed to blend well. Cover and refrigerate from 3 hours to overnight.

Return dough to room temperature. Roll out on a lightly floured board to ¼-inch thickness. Cut with a 2½-inch round cutter or an equivalent cutter. Place on cookie sheets that have been sprayed with cooking spray or lined with aluminum foil.

Bake at 350°F for 10 to 12 minutes, or until cookies are almost firm. Remove cookies to a wire rack and cool to room temperature.

Note: Cookies will be soft if kept in an airtight container. If you want them crisp, freeze them or keep them in a container that isn't airtight.

Yield: 36 cookies
Food exchanges per cookie: 1 starch and 1 fat; or 1 carbohydrate choice
Sugar per cookie: 1.8 teaspoons or 7.5 grams
Low-cholesterol diets: Recipe is suitable as written.
Low-sodium diets: Omit salt. Use salt-free margarine and low-sodium baking powder.
Nutritive values per cookie:

Calories: 115	FAT: 5 g
CHO: 16 g	Na: 98 mg
PRO: 2 g	Cholesterol: 0

Margarine Cookies

These are based on the traditional butter cookies, which are generally shaped with a cookie press or pastry tube. The only difference is that these are made with margarine and the amount of sugar has been reduced.

1 cup (2 sticks) margarine at room temperature	Water as necessary
¾ cup sugar	3 cups all-purpose flour
1½ teaspoons almond extract	1 teaspoon baking soda
2 large eggs	1½ teaspoons cream of tartar
	¼ teaspoon salt

Cream margarine and sugar together at medium speed until light and fluffy. Add flavoring and eggs. (If your 2 eggs don't make ½ cup eggs, add up to 2 tablespoons water for a total of ½ cup eggs and water.) Beat at medium speed for 30 seconds, scraping down the bowl before and after addition. Stir flour, baking soda, cream of tartar, and salt together to blend well; add to creamy mixture. Mix at low speed only until smooth.

Place dough in a cookie press or pastry bag. Form cookies, using 2 teaspoonfuls dough per cookie, on cookie sheets that have been sprayed with cooking spray or lined with aluminum foil.

Bake at 375°F for 10 minutes, or until cookies are lightly browned. Remove them to a wire rack and cool to room temperature.

Yield: 60 cookies
Food exchanges per 2 cookies: 1 starch and 1 fat; or 1 carbohydrate choice
Sugar per 2 cookies: 1.2 teaspoons or 5 grams
Low-cholesterol diets: Omit eggs. Use ½ cup egg whites or liquid egg substitute.
Low-sodium diets: Omit salt. Use salt-free margarine.
Nutritive values per 2 cookies:

Calories: 124	FAT: 7 g
CHO: 15 g	Na: 121 mg
PRO: 2 g	Cholesterol: 18 mg

Spoon River Rolled Cookies

My friend Kay Knochel, of Phoenix, gave me this recipe recently and they are delicious. She got the recipe from lifelong friend Ellsworth Cunningham, whose uncle Lee featured them at his bakery many years ago in London Mills, Illinois, in Spoon River country, which was made famous by Edgar Lee Masters's *Spoon River Anthology*. Kay says people frequently dunked them in coffee.

½ cup vegetable shortening
1¼ cups sugar
2 large eggs
1 teaspoon vanilla
    extract
1 teaspoon lemon extract
3 cups all-purpose flour

1 teaspoon nutmeg
    (optional)
1 teaspoon baking
    powder
1 teaspoon baking soda
¼ teaspoon salt
1 cup sour cream

Cream shortening and sugar together at medium speed until well blended. Add eggs and flavorings, and beat at medium speed until creamy, scraping down the bowl before and after addition. Stir flour, nutmeg if using, baking powder, baking soda, and salt together to blend well; add, along with sour cream, to creamy mixture. Mix at medium speed until smooth and creamy. Cover and refrigerate from 3 hours to overnight.

Return dough to room temperature. Roll out on a lightly floured board to ¼-inch thickness. Cut with a 2½-inch round cutter or an equivalent (see Note below). Place dough on cookie sheets that have been sprayed with cooking spray or lined with aluminum foil.

Bake at 350°F for 8 to 10 minutes, or until cookies are lightly browned. Remove them to a wire rack and cool to room temperature.

Note: Nutritive values for these cookies are based on the use of the 2½-inch round cutter and a weight of a little over 1 ounce per cookie. You may use other cutters as long as the finished cookie weighs about 1 ounce, and you might even make a 2-ounce cookie and figure the nutritive values and exchanges as twice those for the smaller cookie. You may add flavorings other than vanilla and lemon; if you add nuts, raisins and the like, however, you are altering the nutritive values and exchanges for each cookie.

Yield: 36 cookies

Food exchanges per cookie: 1 starch and 1 fat; or 1 carbohydrate choice

Sugar per cookie: 1.7 teaspoons or 7 grams

Low-cholesterol diets: Omit eggs. Use ½ cup egg whites or liquid egg substitute.

Low-sodium diets: Omit salt. Use low-sodium baking powder.

Nutritive values per cookie:

Calories: 108	FAT: 5 g
CHO: 15 g	Na: 54 mg
PRO: 2 g	Cholesterol: 18 mg

Black Walnut Cookies

This recipe is based on one from my friend Vera Wilson. I don't think she recognized it anymore when I got through with it, but she told me she liked my adaptation (before I told her it was based on her recipe!). You may use other types of nuts, if you like, without altering the exchange values.

½ cup (1 stick) margarine at
    room temperature
⅔ cup sugar
Dry sugar substitute equal to
    ¼ cup sugar (optional)
¼ cup egg whites
1 teaspoon vanilla
    extract

1 teaspoon black walnut
    flavoring
¼ cup water
2 cups all-purpose flour
⅓ cup chopped black walnuts
2 tablespoons dry buttermilk
1 teaspoon baking soda
¼ teaspoon salt

Cream margarine, sugar, and dry sugar substitute together at medium speed until light and creamy. Add egg whites, flavorings, and water, and mix at medium speed for 30 seconds, scraping down the bowl before and after addition. Stir flour, walnuts, dry buttermilk, baking soda, and salt together to blend well, and add to creamy mixture. Mix at medium speed to blend. Drop dough by 1½ tablespoonfuls (level no. 40 dipper) onto cookie sheets that have been sprayed with cooking spray or lined with aluminum foil. Press each cookie down to ½-inch thickness with the back of a tablespoon dipped in cold water.

Bake at 350°F for 12 to 14 minutes, or until cookies are browned on the bottom. Remove them to a wire rack and cool to room temperature.

Yield: 24 cookies
Food exchanges per cookie: 1 starch and 1 fat; or 1 carbohydrate
    choice
Sugar per cookie: 1.3 teaspoons or 5 grams
Low-cholesterol diets: Recipe is suitable as written.
Low-sodium diets: Omit salt. Use salt-free margarine.
Nutritive values per cookie:

Calories: 107   FAT: 5 g
CHO: 14 g   Na: 108 mg
PRO: 2 g   Cholesterol: 0

Chocolate Crackle Cookies

I tried rolling these cookies in sugar substitute instead of sugar but I didn't like them as well, and since we can afford the sugar to roll them in, I continue to use it.

²/₃ cup vegetable shortening
²/₃ cup sugar
¼ cup light corn syrup
Dry sugar substitute equal to
¼ cup sugar (optional)
1 large egg
2 teaspoons vanilla extract
2 cups all-purpose flour

½ cup unsweetened
cocoa powder
1½ teaspoons baking
soda
½ teaspoon salt
¼ cup water at room
temperature
¼ cup sugar for rolling

Cream shortening, ²/₃ cup sugar, corn syrup and dry sugar substitute (if using) together at medium speed until light and fluffy. Add egg and vanilla, and beat at medium speed until well blended, scraping down the bowl before and after addition. Stir flour, cocoa, baking soda, and salt together to blend well, and add, along with water, to creamy mixture. Mix at medium speed to blend. Form dough into balls, using 1 tablespoon (level no. 60 dipper) dough per ball. Roll balls in the ¼ cup sugar, and place on cookie sheets that have been sprayed with cooking spray or lined with aluminum foil.

Bake at 350°F for about 12 minutes, or until cookies are almost firm. Remove them to a wire rack and cool to room temperature.

Yield: 30 cookies
Food exchanges per cookie: 1 starch and 1 fat; or 1 carbohydrate choice
Sugar per cookie: 1.5 teaspoons or 6 grams
Low-cholesterol diets: Omit egg. Use ¼ cup egg whites or liquid egg substitute.
Low-sodium diets: Omit salt.
Nutritive values per cookie:

Calories: 106
CHO: 15 g
PRO: 1 g

FAT: 5 g
Na: 81 mg
Cholesterol: 9 mg

Chocolate Dunkin' Cookies

These cookies are for people who want to dunk their cookies efficiently.

½ cup (1 stick) margarine at
   room temperature
¼ cup granulated sugar
¼ cup packed brown sugar
Dry sugar substitute equal to
   ¼ cup sugar
1 teaspoon vanilla extract

½ cup egg whites
2 cups all-purpose flour
¼ cup unsweetened
   cocoa powder
½ teaspoon baking
   soda
¼ teaspoon salt

Cream margarine, sugars, and sugar substitute together until light and fluffy. Add vanilla and egg whites, and mix at medium speed until creamy, scraping down the bowl before and after adding them. Stir flour, cocoa, baking soda, and salt together to blend, and add to creamy mixture. Mix at medium speed to blend. Cover and refrigerate from 1 to 24 hours.

Return dough to room temperature. Roll out on a lightly floured board to form a 12-inch square. Cut dough the long way at 4-inch intervals to make 3 (4 × 12-inch) rectangles. Cut each rectangle into 12 (1 × 4-inch) pieces. Place pieces on cookie sheets that have been sprayed with cooking spray or lined with aluminum foil.

Bake at 350°F for about 10 minutes, or until cookies are firm. Remove them to a wire rack and cool to room temperature.

Variations: Cinnamon Dunkin' Cookies: Omit cocoa. Add ¼ cup all-purpose flour and 1½ teaspoons cinnamon to the flour and other dry ingredients.

Lemon Dunkin' Cookies: Omit cocoa. Add 1 teaspoon lemon flavoring and grated rind from 1 lemon along with the vanilla, and add ¼ cup all-purpose flour to the flour and other dry ingredients.

Yield: 36 cookies
Food exchanges per cookie: 1 starch and 1 fat; or 1 carbohydrate
   choice
Sugar per cookie: 0.7 teaspoon or 3 grams
Low-cholesterol diets: Recipe is suitable as written.
Low-sodium diets: Omit salt. Use salt-free margarine.
Nutritive values per cookie:

Calories: 93	FAT: 4 g
CHO: 13 g	Na: 33 mg
PRO: 2 g	Cholesterol: 0

Chocolate Peanut Cookies

½ cup chunky peanut butter
½ cup (1 stick) margarine at room temperature
1 cup sugar
⅓ cup egg whites
1 teaspoon vanilla extract
1 teaspoon chocolate flavoring (optional)
2 cups all-purpose flour

⅓ cup unsweetened cocoa powder
1 teaspoon baking powder
1 teaspoon baking soda
Dry sugar substitute equal to ¼ cup sugar
¼ teaspoon salt
½ cup chopped roasted peanuts
½ cup coffee at room temperature

Cream peanut butter, margarine, and sugar together at medium speed until light and fluffy. Add egg whites and flavorings, and mix at medium speed for 30 seconds, scraping down the bowl before and after adding them. Stir flour, cocoa, baking powder, baking soda, dry sugar substitute, salt, and peanuts together to blend well. Add flour mixture, along with the coffee, to creamy mixture; mix at medium speed until creamy. Drop dough by 1½ tablespoonfuls (level no. 40 dipper) onto cookie sheets that have been sprayed with cooking spray or lined with aluminum foil. Press each cookie down to ½-inch thickness with the back of a tablespoon dipped in cold water.

Bake at 350°F for about 10 minutes, or until cookies are almost firm. Remove them to a wire rack and cool to room temperature.

Yield: 32 cookies
Food exchanges per cookie: 1 starch and 1 fat; or 1 carbohydrate choice
Sugar per cookie: 1.5 teaspoons or 6 grams
Low-cholesterol diets: Recipe is suitable as written.
Low-sodium diets: Omit salt. Use salt-free margarine, low-sodium peanut butter and baking powder, and unsalted peanuts.
Nutritive values per cookie:

Calories: 118 FAT: 6 g
CHO: 14 g Na: 119 mg
PRO: 3 g Cholesterol: 0

Coconut Cookies

The one-bowl method, which is used frequently for large-quantity recipes, is good for a busy day. It generally produces an excellent cookie, although some cookies have a better texture when you cream the fat and sugar together.

1½ cups all-purpose flour
1 cup sweetened, shredded
  coconut
⅓ cup sugar
¼ teaspoon baking soda
¼ teaspoon salt

½ cup (1 stick) margarine at
  room temperature
¼ cup water
1 large egg
2 teaspoons coconut
  flavoring

Place flour, coconut, sugar, baking soda, and salt in a mixer bowl and mix at low speed until well blended. Add margarine, water, egg, and flavoring, and mix at medium speed to blend. Drop dough by tablespoonfuls (level no. 60 dipper) onto cookie sheets that have been sprayed with cooking spray or lined with aluminum foil. (Cookies will be mounded; if you prefer flat cookies, press each down lightly with the back of a tablespoon dipped in cold water before baking.)

Bake at 375°F for 10 to 12 minutes, or until cookies are browned on the bottom. Remove them to a wire rack and cool to room temperature.

Yield: 24 cookies
Food exchanges per cookie: 1 starch and 1 fat; or 1 carbohydrate
  choice
Sugar per cookie: 1.3 teaspoons or 5 grams
Low-cholesterol diets: Use only ½ cup coconut. Use your discretion in
  deciding to include it in your diet.
Low-sodium diets: Omit salt. Use salt-free margarine.
Nutritive values per cookie:

Calories: 101   FAT: 5 g
CHO: 13 g   Na: 164 mg
PRO: 1 g   Cholesterol: 11 mg

Date Lemon Sugar Cookies

This recipe comes from my friend Jan Franks, of Oelwein, Iowa. It is a soft, flavorful sugar cookie, a good choice for children or anyone who has difficulty chewing a crisp cookie. This cookie is especially delightful accompanied by a cup of hot tea.

1/3 cup margarine at room temperature

1/3 cup sugar

2 teaspoons lemon extract

1/4 cup egg whites or liquid egg substitute

1 tablespoon unsweetened applesauce

2 tablespoons lemon juice

2 tablespoons grated fresh or finely chopped dried lemon rind

2 1/4 cups all-purpose flour

1/2 teaspoon baking soda

1/2 cup chopped dates

1/2 cup water at room temperature

Using an electric mixer at medium speed, cream margarine, sugar, and lemon extract together until light and fluffy. Add egg whites or liquid egg substitute, applesauce, lemon juice, and lemon rind and mix at medium speed for 30 seconds, scraping down the bowl before and after the addition.

Stir flour, baking soda, and dates together to blend and add, along with the water, to the egg mixture. Mix at medium speed to blend. Drop the dough by 1 1/2 tablespoonfuls (level no. 40 dipper) onto cookie sheets that have been sprayed with cooking spray or lined with aluminum foil. Using the back of a tablespoon dipped in cold water, gently press each cookie down to about 1/2 inch-thickness.

Bake in a 350°F oven for 10 to 12 minutes, or until lightly browned and firm. Cool on wire racks.

Yield: 30 cookies
Food exchanges per cookie: 1 starch; or 1 carbohydrate choice
Sugar per cookie: 1.2 teaspoons or 5 grams
Low-cholesterol diets: Recipe is suitable as written.
Low-sodium diets: Use salt-free margarine.
Nutritive values per cookie:

Calories: 64
CHO: 11 g
PRO: 2 g
FAT: 2 g
Na: 48 mg
Cholesterol: 0

Double Chocolate Cookies

1 cup 100% Bran, Bran Buds, or All Bran
1/3 cup water
2 large eggs
2 teaspoons vanilla extract
1/3 cup vegetable oil
Dry sugar substitute equal to 1/2 cup sugar
1 cup all-purpose flour

1/3 cup unsweetened cocoa powder
2 tablespoons instant nonfat dry milk
1/2 teaspoon baking soda
1/2 teaspoon baking powder
1/4 teaspoon salt
1/4 teaspoon cinnamon
1/2 cup sugar
1/2 cup miniature semisweet chocolate chips

Place cereal, water, eggs, vanilla, oil, and sugar substitute in mixer bowl and stir lightly until blended. Let mixture set for 30 minutes.

In another bowl, stir together flour, cocoa, dry milk, baking soda, baking powder, salt, cinnamon, and sugar to blend well. Add to the bran mixture. Beat at medium speed to blend. Stir in the chocolate chips. Drop dough by 1 1/2 tablespoonfuls (level no. 40 dipper) onto cookie sheets that have been sprayed with cooking spray or lined with aluminum foil.

Bake at 350°F for 10 to 12 minutes, or until firm. Do not overbake. Remove to wire rack and cool to room temperature.

Yield: 24 cookies
Food exchanges per cookie: 1 starch and 1 fat; or 1 carbohydrate choice
Sugar per cookie: 1.7 teaspoons or 7 grams
Low-cholesterol diets: Omit eggs. Use 1/2 cup egg whites or liquid egg substitute.
Low-sodium diets: Omit salt. Use low-sodium baking powder.
Nutritive values per cookie:

Calories: 110   FAT: 4.5 g
CHO: 18 g   Na: 85 mg
PRO: 2 g   Cholesterol: 20 mg

Drop Sugar Cookies

These crisp sugar cookies can be tinted with food coloring for special occasions. They can also be topped with almond, pecan, or walnut halves.

1 cup granulated sugar
1 cup powdered sugar
1 cup (2 sticks) margarine at room temperature
¾ cup vegetable oil
½ cup egg whites or liquid egg substitute, at room temperature

1 teaspoon vanilla extract
4½ cups all-purpose flour
1 teaspoon baking soda
1 teaspoon cream of tartar

Place sugars, margarine, and oil in the bowl of an electric mixer and mix at medium speed until creamy. Add egg whites or liquid egg substitute and vanilla and mix at medium speed until creamy, scraping the bowl before and after the addition.

Stir flour, baking soda, and cream of tartar together to blend and add to the creamy mixture and mix at medium speed until smooth. Drop the dough by 1 tablespoonful (level no. 60 dipper) onto cookie sheets that have been sprayed with cooking spray or lined with aluminum foil. Gently press each cookie down lightly with the back of a tablespoon dipped in cold water.

Bake at 375°F for 12 to 15 minutes, or until lightly browned around the edges. Cool on wire racks.

Variations: Black Walnut Drop Sugar Cookies: Add 1 teaspoon black walnut flavoring with the vanilla and ¾ cup chopped black walnuts with the flour mixture.

Raisin Drop Sugar Cookies: Add ¾ cup chopped raisins with the flour mixture.

Candied Fruit Drop Sugar Cookies: Add ¾ cup chopped candied fruit with the flour mixture.

Lemon Drop Sugar Cookies: Omit vanilla and add 2 teaspoons lemon extract and 1 tablespoon finely chopped fresh or dried lemon peel.

Yield: 72 cookies
Food exchanges per cookie: ½ starch and 1 fat; or 1 carbohydrate choice
Sugar per cookie: 1.3 teaspoons or 5.3 grams
Low-cholesterol diets: Recipe is suitable as written.
Low-sodium diets: Use salt-free margarine.
Nutritive values per cookie:

Calories: 88
CHO: 10 g
PRO: 1 g

FAT: 5 g
Na: 44 mg
Cholesterol: 0

Germantown Cookies

⅔ cup (1⅓ sticks) margarine at room temperature
½ cup granulated sugar
½ cup packed brown sugar
¼ cup unsweetened applesauce
⅓ cup egg whites or liquid egg substitute

1 teaspoon vanilla extract
2¼ cups all-purpose flour
¾ teaspoon baking powder
¾ teaspoon baking soda
1 cup rolled oats

Using an electric mixer at medium speed, cream margarine and sugars together until light and fluffy. Add applesauce, egg whites or liquid egg substitute, and vanilla. Mix at medium speed until creamy, scraping down the bowl before and after addition.

Stir flour, baking powder, baking soda, and oats together to blend and add to the creamy mixture. Mix at medium speed until well blended. Drop the dough by 1½ tablespoonfuls (level no. 40 dipper) onto cookie sheets that have been sprayed with cooking spray or lined with aluminum foil.

Bake at 350°F for 15 minutes, or until almost firm. Cool on wire racks.

Yield: 42 cookies
Food exchanges per cookie: 1 starch; or 1 carbohydrate choice
Sugar per cookie: 1.2 teaspoons or 5 grams
Low-cholesterol diets: Recipe is suitable as written.
Low-sodium diets: Use salt-free margarine and low-sodium baking powder.
Nutritive values per cookie:

Calories: 78
CHO: 12 g
PRO: 1 g

FAT: 3 g
Na: 69 mg
Cholesterol: 0

Cornish Cookies

This recipe is based on one from my friend Margaret Foxwell, of Elgin, Iowa. Her recipe came from her husband's family, who came from Cornwall, in southwestern England, and settled in Iowa in the mid-1800s.

½ cup packed brown sugar
Dry brown sugar substitute
   equal to ½ cup brown sugar
½ cup (1 stick) margarine at
   room temperature
¼ cup molasses

1 large egg
1 teaspoon vinegar
2¼ cups all-purpose flour
1½ teaspoons baking soda
½ teaspoon ginger
½ teaspoon cinnamon

Combine brown sugar, dry brown sugar substitute, margarine, and molasses in a mixer bowl and mix at medium speed until creamy. Add egg and vinegar, and mix at medium speed for 30 seconds, scraping down the bowl before and after addition. Stir flour, baking soda, ginger, and cinnamon together to blend well, and add to creamy mixture. Mix at medium speed to blend. Form dough into balls, using 1 tablespoon (level no. 60 dipper) dough per ball. Place balls on cookie sheets that have been sprayed with cooking spray or lined with aluminum foil. Press balls down to ½-inch thickness with the back of a tablespoon dipped in cold water.

Bake at 350°F for about 15 minutes, or until cookies are lightly browned and firm. Remove them to a wire rack and cool to room temperature.

Yield: 24 cookies
Food exchanges per cookie: 1 starch and 1 fat; or 1 carbohydrate
   choice
Sugar per cookie: 1.5 teaspoons or 6 grams
Low-cholesterol diets: Omit egg. Use ¼ cup egg whites or liquid egg
   substitute.
Low-sodium diets: Use salt-free margarine.
Nutritive values per cookie:

Calories: 104
CHO: 15 g
PRO: 2 g

FAT: 4 g
Na: 119 mg
Cholesterol: 11 mg

Sour Cream–Ginger Cookies

¼ cup vegetable oil
½ cup packed brown
  sugar
⅓ cup molasses
1 large egg
½ cup sour cream

2 cups all-purpose flour
½ teaspoon baking soda
½ teaspoon ginger
½ teaspoon cinnamon
½ teaspoon cloves
½ teaspoon salt

Place oil, brown sugar, molasses, egg, and sour cream in a mixer bowl and mix at medium speed to blend well. Stir flour, baking soda, ginger, cinnamon, cloves, and salt together to blend well, and add to sour cream mixture. Mix at medium speed until creamy. Drop dough by 1½ tablespoonfuls (level no. 40 dipper) onto cookie sheets that have been sprayed with cooking spray or lined with aluminum foil.

Bake at 375°F for about 10 minutes, or until cookies are firm and lightly browned. Remove them to a wire rack and cool to room temperature.

Yield: 24 cookies
Food exchanges per cookie: 1 starch and 1 fat; or 1 carbohydrate
  choice
Sugar per cookie: Equivalent to 1.7 teaspoons or 7 grams
Low-cholesterol diets: Omit egg. Use ¼ cup egg whites or liquid egg
  substitute.
Low-sodium diets: Omit salt.
Nutritive values per cookie:

Calories: 92	FAT: 4 g
CHO: 15 g	Na: 90 mg
PRO: 1 g	Cholesterol: 14 mg

Hermits

Many people think of this as a recipe from New England, but these cookies are popular all over the country. Perhaps we should think of them as all-American.

½ cup (1 stick) margarine at room temperature
⅔ cup packed brown sugar
2 large eggs
2 cups all-purpose flour
1 teaspoon baking powder
¼ teaspoon salt

Dry sugar substitute equal to ¼ cup sugar (optional)
1 teaspoon cinnamon
½ teaspoon nutmeg
¼ teaspoon ginger
¼ cup chopped walnuts
¼ cup raisins
¼ cup water at room temperature

Cream margarine and brown sugar together at medium speed until light and fluffy. Add eggs and mix at medium speed for 1 minute, scraping down the bowl before and after addition. Stir flour, baking powder, salt, dry sugar substitute (if using), cinnamon, nutmeg, ginger, walnuts, and raisins together to blend well. Add, along with water, to creamy mixture; mix at medium speed to blend well. Drop dough by 1½ tablespoonfuls (level no. 40 dipper) onto cookie sheets that have been sprayed with cooking spray or lined with aluminum foil.

Bake at 350°F for 10 to 12 minutes, or until cookies are browned on the bottom. Remove them to a wire rack and cool to room temperature.

Yield: 24 cookies
Food exchanges per cookie: 1 starch and 1 fat; or 1 carbohydrate choice
Sugar per cookie: 1.3 teaspoons or 5 grams
Low-cholesterol diets: Omit eggs. Use ½ cup egg whites or liquid egg substitute.
Low-sodium diets: Omit salt. Use salt-free margarine and low-sodium baking powder.
Nutritive values per cookie:

Calories: 114
CHO: 15 g
PRO: 2 g

FAT: 5 g
Na: 89 mg
Cholesterol: 23 mg

Honey Cookies

These cookies are a favorite of Dad's cousin, Vera Kriener, of Waucoma, Iowa. I've modified them a bit to lower the sugar but keep the great taste. This recipe does not have eggs. It is very moist and the cookies keep well in a tightly covered container. It's a big recipe, so you might want to cut it in half.

1 cup (2 sticks) margarine at room temperature
¾ cup sugar, plus ¼ cup for dipping
¾ cup honey
1 tablespoon vanilla extract

5 cups all-purpose flour
1 tablespoon baking soda
¼ teaspoon cinnamon
¼ teaspoon ginger
½ cup cold water

Beat margarine, ¾ cup sugar, honey, and vanilla at medium speed until light and fluffy. Stir flour, baking soda, cinnamon, and ginger together. Add to creamy mixture alternately with cold water. Shape into a ball, cover with plastic wrap, and refrigerate until chilled.

Form dough into balls using 1½ tablespoonfuls (level no. 40 dipper). Dip balls in remaining ¼ cup sugar. Place onto cookie sheets that have been sprayed with cooking spray or lined with aluminum foil. Using the back of a tablespoon dipped in cold water, gently flatten slightly.

Bake at 350°F for about 10 minutes, or until golden brown. Watch carefully so as not to overbake.

Yield: 66 cookies
Food exchanges per cookie: 1 starch; or 1 carbohydrate choice
Sugar per cookie: 1.2 teaspoons or 5 grams
Low cholesterol diets: Recipe is suitable as written.
Low sodium diets: Recipe is suitable as written.
Nutritive values per cookie:

Calories: 80
CHO: 13 g
PRO: 1 g

FAT: 3 g
Na: 89 mg
Cholesterol: 0

Iowa Pride Cookies

I modified these cookies from a favorite recipe of my husband's aunt, Rose Catherine Schulte, of Waukon, Iowa.

¾ cup packed brown sugar	1 teaspoon baking soda
¾ cup granulated sugar	1 teaspoon baking powder
1 cup (2 sticks) margarine at room temperatue	⅛ teaspoon cinnamon
	½ cup sweetened, shredded
2 large eggs	coconut
½ teaspoon vanilla extract	1⅓ cups rolled oats
1 cup all-purpose flour	½ cup Kellog's Rice Krispies

Beat sugars and margarine at medium speed until light and fluffy. Add eggs and vanilla and beat until well mixed. Stir together flour, baking soda, baking powder, cinnamon, coconut, oats, and cereal.

Form dough into balls using 1½ tablespoonfuls (level no. 40 dipper) and place on ungreased cookie sheet.

Bake at 350°F for 12 to 15 minutes, or until light brown. Watch carefully so you do not overbake or cookies will be too crisp.

Yield: 48 cookies
Food exchanges per cookie: 1 starch; or 1 carbohydrate choice
Sugar per cookie: 2.2 teaspoons or 9 grams
Low-cholesterol diet: Omit eggs. Use ½ cup liquid egg substitute.
Low-sodium diet: Use low-sodium baking powder.
Nutritive values per cookie:

Calories: 90	FAT: 4 g
CHO: 13 g	Na: 97 mg
PRO: .7 g	Cholesterol: 4.5 mg

Lemon Cookies

These are my sister Shirley's favorite cookies. They have a wonderful lemony taste and are easy to make. The recipe is correct even though there does seem to be too much sugar in it.

¾ cup sugar
½ cup dry lemonade mix
  (not sugar-free)
¼ cup light corn syrup
¾ cup (1½ sticks) margarine at
  room temperature

¼ cup egg whites
2¼ cups all-purpose
  flour
½ teaspoon baking
  soda

Cream sugar, lemonade mix, corn syrup, and margarine together at medium speed until light and fluffy. Add egg whites and mix at medium speed until smooth, scraping down the bowl before and after adding them. Stir flour and baking soda together to blend, and then add to creamy mixture. Mix at medium speed to blend. Drop dough by tablespoonfuls (level no. 60 dipper) onto cookie sheets that have been sprayed with cooking spray or lined with aluminum foil.

Bake at 350°F for 8 to 10 minutes, or until cookies are browned on the bottom. Remove them to a wire rack and cool to room temperature.

Yield: 36 cookies
Food exchanges per cookie: 1 starch and 1 fat; or 1 carbohydrate
  choice
Sugar per cookie: 2 teaspoons or 8 grams
Low-cholesterol diets: Recipe is suitable as written.
Low-sodium diets: Use salt-free margarine.
Nutritive values per cookie:

Calories: 96
CHO: 15 g
PRO: 1 g

FAT: 4 g
Na: 60 mg
Cholesterol: 0

Lemon Licorice Cookies

If you don't like anise seed in your cookies, you can use 1 teaspoon of anise flavoring instead of the anise seeds, with no change in the food exchanges.

¾ cup (1½ sticks) margarine at room temperature
¾ cup dry lemonade mix (not sugar-free)
¼ cup sugar
1 tablespoon anise seed

¼ cup water
¼ cup egg whites
3 cups all-purpose flour
¼ cup instant nonfat dry milk
1 teaspoon baking soda
½ teaspoon salt

Cream margarine, lemonade mix, sugar, and anise seed together at medium speed until light and fluffy. Add water and egg whites, and mix at medium speed for 30 seconds, scraping down the bowl before and after addition. Stir flour, dry milk, soda, and salt together to blend well, and add to creamy mixture. Mix at medium speed to blend. Drop dough by 1½ tablespoonfuls (level no. 40 dipper) onto cookie sheets that have been sprayed with cooking spray or lined with aluminum foil. Press each cookie down lightly with the back of a tablespoon dipped in cold water.

Bake at 350°F for 12 to 15 minutes, or until cookies are lightly browned. Remove them to a wire rack and cool to room temperature.

Yield: 36 cookies
Food exchanges per cookie: 1 starch and 1 fat; or 1 carbohydrate choice
Sugar per cookie: 1.3 teaspoons or 5.5 grams
Low-cholesterol diets: Recipe is suitable as written.
Low-sodium diets: Omit salt. Use salt-free margarine.
Nutritive values per cookie:

Calories: 91
CHO: 14 g
PRO: 2 g

FAT: 4 g
Na: 111 mg
Cholesterol: 0

Crunch Molasses Cookies

These delicious cookies have a delicate taste of ginger and molasses—perfect on an autumn day. They are a family favorite from Mabel's mom's cookbook.

2 cups sifted all-purpose flour	½ cup vegetable shortening
2 teaspoons baking powder	¼ cup packed brown sugar
½ teaspoon cloves	½ cup granulated sugar, plus
½ teaspoon ginger	extra for coating
1 teaspoon cinnamon	1 large egg
¼ teaspoon salt	¼ cup dark molasses

Sift together flour, baking powder, spices, and salt and set aside. Beat shortening and sugars on medium speed until light and fluffy. Add egg and mix well. Add molasses and flour mixture, ⅓ at a time, and mix well.

Form dough into balls using 1 tablespoonful (level no. 60 dipper) and roll in granulated sugar. Place 2 inches apart on cookie sheet that has been sprayed with cooking spray.

Bake at 350°F for 15 minutes, or until browned.

Note: Do not bake on bottom rack of oven as they burn easily.

Yield: 54 cookies
Food exchanges per cookie: 1 starch and 1 fat; or 1 carbohydrate choice
Sugar per cookie: 2 teaspoons or 8 grams
Low-cholesterol diets: Omit egg. Use ¼ cup liquid egg substitute.
Low-sodium diets: Omit salt. Use low-sodium baking powder.
Nutritive values per cookie:

Calories: 100	FAT: 4 g
CHO: 14 g	Na: 100 mg
PRO: 2 g	Cholesterol: 10 mg

Dick's Molasses Cookies

These cookies are a favorite of my cousin Virginia Ballantine and her family. Her husband, Dick, who is retired, makes dozens of them when their grandchildren come for a visit. You can bake them without rolling them in sugar first; they don't look as good that way—but they're just as delicious.

¾ cup sugar, plus ¼ cup for rolling
¼ cup molasses
¾ cup (1½ sticks) margarine at room temperature
¼ cup egg whites at room temperature

2¼ cups all-purpose flour
2 teaspoons baking soda
1 teaspoon cinnamon
¼ teaspoon ginger

Cream ¾ cup of the sugar, molasses, and margarine together at medium speed until creamy. Add egg whites and mix at medium speed until creamy, scraping down the bowl before and after addition. Stir flour, baking soda, cinnamon, and ginger together to blend well. Add to creamy mixture and mix at medium speed to blend well. Form dough into balls, using 1 tablespoon (level no. 60 dipper) dough per ball. Roll balls in remaining ¼ cup sugar (I use a bowl containing ½ cup sugar to make coating easier but use only ¼ cup of it for the cookies), and place on cookie sheets that have been sprayed with cooking spray or lined with aluminum foil.

Bake at 350°F for 8 to 10 minutes, or until cookies are firm. Leave them on sheets for 2 to 3 minutes; then remove cookies to a wire rack and cool to room temperature.

Yield: 36 cookies
Food exchanges per cookie: 1 starch and 1 fat; or 1 carbohydrate choice
Sugar per cookie: 1.3 teaspoons or 5.5 grams
Low-cholesterol diets: Recipe is suitable as written. Low-sodium diets: Use salt-free margarine.
Nutritive values per cookie:

Calories: 89
CHO: 13 g
PRO: 1 g

FAT: 4 g
Na: 95 mg
Cholesterol: 0

Soft Molasses Cookies

These soft cookies have an excellent flavor.

1/4 cup sugar
3/4 cup molasses
1/2 cup vegetable shortening
2 large eggs
2 3/4 cups all-purpose flour
2 teaspoons baking soda
1 teaspoon cinnamon

1 teaspoon ginger
1/2 teaspoon nutmeg
1/2 teaspoon salt
Dry sugar substitute equal to 1/4 cup sugar
1/2 cup hot coffee
1 tablespoon lemon juice

Cream sugar, molasses, and shortening together at medium speed until light and fluffy. Add eggs and mix at medium speed until creamy, scraping down the bowl before and after addition. Stir flour, baking soda, cinnamon, ginger, nutmeg, salt, and dry sugar substitute together to blend well, and then add, along with coffee and lemon juice, to creamy mixture. Mix at medium speed until creamy. Drop dough by 1 1/2 tablespoonfuls (level no. 40 dipper) onto cookie sheets that have been sprayed with cooking spray or lined with aluminum foil.

Bake at 375°F for 12 to 14 minutes, or until cookies are firm. Remove them to a wire rack and cool to room temperature.

Yield: 30 cookies
Food exchanges per cookie: 1 starch and 1 fat; or 1 carbohydrate choice
Sugar per cookie: Equivalent to 1.6 teaspoons or 7 grams
Low-cholesterol diets: Omit eggs. Use 1/2 cup egg whites or liquid egg substitute.
Low-sodium diets: Omit salt.
Nutritive values per cookie:

Calories: 101
CHO: 15 g
PRO: 2 g

FAT: 4 g
Na: 103 mg
Cholesterol: 18 mg

Monster Cookies

This recipe is a favorite of Anna Daab, of Holland, Michigan. Anna is a very lucky little girl. Her mother develops wonderful recipes for her, and her father and two brothers are also very supportive of her and her need to remain a normal little girl who just happens to have diabetes.

¾ cup egg whites
¾ cup packed brown sugar
½ cup granulated sugar
1 cup crunchy peanut butter
1 teaspoon vanilla extract

⅓ cup vegetable oil
4 cups rolled oats
1 teaspoon baking soda
½ cup semisweet chocolate
    chips

Place egg whites, sugars, peanut butter, vanilla, and oil in a mixer bowl and mix at medium speed to blend well. Add oats, baking soda, and chocolate chips to creamy mixture and mix at medium speed to blend. Drop dough by 1½ tablespoonfuls (level no. 40 dipper) onto cookie sheets that have been sprayed with cooking spray or lined with aluminum foil. Press each cookie down lightly to ½-inch thickness with the back of a tablespoon dipped in cold water.

Bake at 350°F for 12 minutes, or until cookies are lightly browned and firm. Remove them to a wire rack and cool to room temperature.

Yield: 36 cookies
Food exchanges per cookie: 1 starch and 1 fat; or 1 carbohydrate choice
Sugar per cookie: 1.7 teaspoons or 7 grams
Low-cholesterol diets: Recipe is suitable as written.
Low-sodium diets: Use low-sodium peanut butter.
Nutritive values per cookie:

Calories: 137
CHO: 16 g
PRO: 4 g

FAT: 7 g
Na: 44 mg
Cholesterol: 0

Orange Tea Cookies

This is another recipe from my friend Diane Daab, of Holland, Michigan.

1 cup sugar
1/3 cup vegetable oil
2/3 cup plain low-fat yogurt
1/4 cup egg whites
1 teaspoon orange flavoring
2 tablespoons thawed, unsweetened frozen orange juice concentrate

3 teaspoons grated fresh or chopped dried orange rind
Dry sugar substitute equal to 1/4 cup sugar
2 1/4 cups all-purpose flour
1/2 teaspoon baking soda
1/2 teaspoon baking powder

Frosting

1/4 cup powdered sugar
2 tablespoons margarine at room temperature

1 1/2 tablespoons thawed orange juice concentrate
1 teaspoon orange rind

Place sugar, oil, yogurt, egg whites, flavoring, orange juice concentrate, rind, and sugar substitute in a mixer bowl and mix at medium speed until creamy. Stir flour, baking soda, and baking powder together to blend, and add to creamy mixture. Mix until creamy. Drop dough by tablespoonfuls (level no. 60 dipper) onto cookie sheets that have been sprayed with cooking spray or lined with aluminum foil.

Bake at 375°F for 15 minutes, or until cookies are lightly browned. Remove them to a wire rack and cool to room temperature.

For frosting: Stir powdered sugar, margarine, orange juice concentrate, and rind together to form a frosting. Frost cooled cookies, using 1/2 teaspoon frosting per cookie.

Yield: 36 cookies
Food exchanges per cookie: 1 starch and 1/2 fat; or 1 carbohydrate choice
Sugar per cookie: 1.3 teaspoons or 5 grams
Low-cholesterol diets: Recipe is suitable as written.
Low-sodium diets: Use salt-free margarine and low-sodium baking powder.
Nutritive values per cookie:

Calories: 87	FAT: 3 g
CHO: 14 g	Na: 29 mg
PRO: 1 g	Cholesterol: 0

Double Peanut Cookies

If you like peanuts and peanut butter, you'll love these cookies, which combine both of them.

¼ cup (½ stick) margarine at room temperature	¼ cup water
1 cup sugar	1¼ cups all-purpose flour
½ cup peanut butter	½ teaspoon baking soda
1 teaspoon vanilla extract	½ teaspoon salt
	1 cup chopped roasted peanuts

Cream margarine, sugar, and peanut butter together until light and fluffy. Add vanilla and water, and mix at medium speed for 1 minute. Stir flour, baking soda, salt, and peanuts together and add to creamy mixture. Mix at medium speed to blend. Drop dough by 1½ tablespoonfuls (level no. 40 dipper) onto cookie sheets that have been sprayed with cooking spray or lined with aluminum foil.

Bake at 350°F for 12 minutes, or until cookies are lightly browned. Leave them on sheets for about 3 minutes, then remove cookies to a wire rack and cool to room temperature.

Yield: 24 cookies

Food exchanges per cookie: 1 starch and 1½ fat; or 1 carbohydrate choice

Sugar per cookie: 2 teaspoons or 8 grams

Low-cholesterol diets: Recipe is suitable as written.

Low-sodium diets: Omit salt. Use salt-free margarine, low-sodium peanut butter, and unsalted peanuts.

Nutritive values per cookie:

Calories: 137	FAT: 8 g
CHO: 15 g	Na: 135 mg
PRO: 4 g	Cholesterol: 0

Pizzelles

3 large eggs
1/3 cup sugar
1 1/2 teaspoons vanilla extract
1/2 cup margarine, melted and cooled (Do not use oil.)

1 cup all-purpose flour
1/2 teaspoon baking powder
1/4 cup ground nuts (optional)

Beat eggs at medium speed until light. Gradually beat in sugar. Add vanilla and margarine to the egg mixture and beat until blended.

Stir flour, baking powder, and nuts (if using) together. Add to egg mixture and stir until smooth. Preheat pizzelle iron according to manufacturer's directions. Drop dough by spoon onto hot pizzelle iron and bake according to directions.

Yield: 20 cookies
Food exchanges per cookie: 1/2 starch and 1 fat; or 1/2 carbohydrate choice
Sugar per cookie: .7 teaspoon or 3 grams
Low-cholesterol diets: Omit eggs. Use 3/4 cup liquid egg substitute.
Low-sodium diets: Use low-sodium baking powder and salt-free margarine.
Nutritive values per cookie:

Calories: 84
CHO: 8 g
PRO: 2 g

FAT: 5 g
Na: 56 mg
Cholesterol: 35 mg

Pumpkin Pillows

½ cup vegetable shortening
1 cup packed brown sugar
2 large eggs
1 teaspoon lemon juice
1 teaspoon vanilla extract
¼ cup canned solid pack
  pumpkin

1½ cups all-purpose
  flour
1 teaspoon baking powder
1 teaspoon baking soda
1½ teaspoons pumpkin pie
  spice
½ cup chopped pecans

Cream shortening and brown sugar together at medium speed until light and fluffy. Add eggs, lemon juice, vanilla, and pumpkin, and mix at medium speed until creamy, scraping down the bowl before and after adding them. Stir flour, baking powder, baking soda, spice, and pecans together and add to creamy mixture. Mix at medium speed until creamy. Drop dough by tablespoonfuls (level no. 60 dipper) onto cookie sheets that have been sprayed with cooking spray or lined with aluminum foil.

Bake at 350°F for 12 to 14 minutes, or until cookies are firm and lightly browned on the bottom. Remove them to a wire rack and cool to room temperature.

Yield: 30 cookies

Food exchanges per cookie: 1 starch and 1 fat; or 1 carbohydrate choice

Sugar per cookie: 1.6 teaspoons or 7 grams

Low-cholesterol diets: Omit eggs. Use ½ cup egg whites or liquid egg substitute.

Low-sodium diets: Use low-sodium baking powder.

Nutritive values per cookie:

Calories: 100	FAT: 5 g
CHO: 13 g	Na: 47 mg
PRO: 1 g	Cholesterol: 18 mg

Pumpkin Spice Cookies

I like to serve these soft, spicy cookies in the fall with a pitcher of apple cider.

½ cup (1 stick) margarine at room temperature
¾ cup packed brown sugar
½ cup egg whites or liquid egg substitute
1 teaspoon maple flavoring
¾ cup canned solid pack pumpkin

1½ cups all-purpose flour
1 teaspoon baking powder
½ teaspoon baking soda
1 teaspoon pumpkin pie spice
1 teaspoon cinnamon
½ cup raisins

Using an electric mixer at medium speed, cream margarine and brown sugar until light and fluffy. Add egg whites or liquid egg substitute, maple flavoring, and pumpkin and mix at medium speed until creamy, scraping the bowl before and after the addition.

Stir flour, baking powder, baking soda, pumpkin pie spice, cinnamon, and raisins together and add to the creamy mixture. Mix to blend. Drop dough by 1½ tablespoonfuls (level no. 40 dipper) onto cookie sheets that have been sprayed with cooking spray or lined with aluminum foil.

Bake at 350°F for 15 minutes or until firm. Cool on wire racks. Makes 30 cookies.

Variation: M&Ms Pumpkin Spice Cookies: Omit the raisins and add 1 fall color M&Ms candy to the top of each cookie.

Yield: 30 cookies
Food exchanges per cookie: 1 starch; or 1 carbohydrate choice
Sugar per cookie: 1.7 teaspoons or 7 grams
Low-cholesterol diets: Recipe is suitable as written.
Low-sodium diets: Use salt-free margarine and low-sodium baking powder.
Nutritive values per cookie:

Calories: 80
CHO: 12 g
PRO: 1 g

FAT: 3 g
Na: 95 mg
Cholesterol: 0

Scottish Shortbread

One Christmas I made these cookies in 5 × 3-inch rectangles then wrote the names of each of our guests on them in frosting. Everyone loved these edible place cards, especially the children.

1¼ cups margarine at room temperature
¾ cup sugar
2 tablespoons unsweetened applesauce

1 teaspoon vanilla or almond extract
3 cups all-purpose flour

Using an electric mixer set at medium speed, cream margarine, sugar, applesauce, and vanilla or almond extract together until light and fluffy. Scrape down the bowl, add flour, and mix at medium speed to form a stiff dough.

Turn the dough out onto a lightly floured board, knead lightly, and roll out to ¼-inch thickness. Using a 2½-inch square cookie cutter, cut dough into squares. Place squares on cookie sheets that have been sprayed with cooking spray or lined with aluminum foil.

Bake at 350°F for 18 to 20 minutes, or until lightly browned on the bottoms. Cool on wire racks.

Variation: Whole-Wheat Shortbread: Substitute ¾ cup packed brown sugar for the sugar. Use 1½ cups all-purpose flour and 1½ cups whole-wheat flour instead of 3 cups all-purpose flour.

Yield: 42 cookies
Food exchanges per cookie: 1 starch; or 1 carbohydrate choice
Sugar per cookie: 1 teaspoon or 4 grams
Low-cholesterol diets: Recipe is suitable as written.
Low-sodium diets: Recipe is suitable as written.
Nutritive values per cookie:

Calories: 90
CHO: 11 g
PRO: 1 g

FAT: 5 g
Na: 65 mg
Cholesterol: 0

Sour Cream Cookies

I modified these sour cream cookies from my sister-in-law Kristin Kriener, of Britt, Iowa. With or without the frosting, these cookies are scrumptious. They are so good, they seldom make it into the cookie jar.

¾ cup butter or margarine at room temperature
1¾ cups packed brown sugar
2 eggs
1½ teaspoons vanilla extract
1 cup light sour cream (reserve 3 tablespoons for frosting, below)

4 cups all-purpose flour
1½ teaspoons baking soda
1½ teaspoons baking powder
½ teaspoon salt
1 cup cashews (optional)

Beat butter or margarine at medium speed until smooth. Add the brown sugar and beat until light and fluffy. Beat in the eggs, one at a time. Add the vanilla and sour cream and mix well. Stir flour, baking soda, baking powder, and salt to blend. Stir flour mixture into creamy mixture until combined. Mix in the cashews (if using).

Refrigerate the dough for at least 1 hour. Drop dough by 1½ table-spoonfuls (level no. 40 dipper) onto ungreased cookie sheets.

Bake at 325°F for 10 minutes, or until very light brown. Allow cookies to cool. Frost if desired. Makes 60 cookies.

Yield: 60 cookies
Food exchanges per cookie: 1 starch and 1 fruit; or 1 carbohydrate choice
Sugar per cookie: 1.7 teaspoons or 7 grams
Low-cholesterol diets: Use margarine. Omit eggs. Use ½ cup egg whites or liquid egg substitute. May use fat-free sour cream if desired.
Low-sodium diets: Omit the salt. Use low-sodium baking powder and salt-free margarine.
Nutritive values per cookie:

Calories: 139	FAT: 3 g
CHO: 13 g	Na: 103 mg
PRO: 1 g	Cholesterol: 14 mg

Sour Cream Frosting

⅓ cup butter at room temperature
3 tablespoons light sour cream (reserved from cookies)

1 teaspoon vanilla extract
2 cups powdered sugar
Fat-free milk as needed

Cream butter, sour cream, and vanilla together until light and fluffy. Add powdered sugar and mix until smooth. If necessary, thin with 1 to 2 teaspoons of fat-free milk. Frost cookies lightly after they have cooled. Enough frosting for 60 cookies.

Yield: 60 frosted cookies

Food exchanges per cookie: 1½ starch and 1 fat; or 1 carbohydrate choice

Sugar per cookie: 2.4 teaspoons or 10 grams

Low-cholesterol diets: Use margarine instead of butter. Use fat-free sour cream if desired.

Low-sodium diets: Omit the salt. Use low-sodium baking powder and salt-free margarine.

Nutritive values per frosted cookie:

Calories: 167	FAT: 5 g
CHO: 16 g	Na: 115 mg
PRO: 1 g	Cholesterol: 18 mg

Swedish Almond Crescents

These delicate cookies are festive at the holidays or any time of year.

1/3 cup margarine
1/4 cup sugar
2 tablespoons unsweetened applesauce
1/2 teaspoon almond extract

1²/3 cups all-purpose flour
1/2 cup ground or very finely chopped almonds
1/4 cup water
1/4 cup powdered sugar

Using an electric mixer at medium speed, beat margarine, sugar, applesauce, and almond extract until light and fluffy. Add flour, almonds, and water to the creamy mixture and mix at medium speed to blend.

Turn dough out onto a lightly floured board, knead lightly, and divide into 24 portions of 1 tablespoon each (level no. 60 dipper). Shape each portion into a roll about 4 inches long with tapered ends. Form the rolls into crescents and place them on cookie sheets that have been sprayed with cooking spray or lined with aluminum foil.

Bake at 375°F for 8 to 10 minutes, or until lightly browned on the bottoms. Dredge warm crescents in powdered sugar and place on wire racks and cool to room temperature. Store in an airtight container or freeze until needed. Makes 24 crescents.

Variation: Black Walnut Crescents: Omit almond extract and almonds. Add 1/2 teaspoon black walnut flavoring and 2/3 cup finely chopped black walnuts.

Yield: 24 cookies
Food exchanges per cookie: 1 starch; or 1 carbohydrate choice
Sugar per cookie: 0.75 teaspoon or 3 grams
Low-cholesterol diets: Recipe is suitable as written.
Low-sodium diets: Use salt-free margarine.
Nutritive values per cookie:

Calories: 80
CHO: 10 g
PRO: 2 g

FAT: 4 g
Na: 30 mg
Cholesterol: 0

Viennese Crescents

1¾ cups all-purpose flour
2 tablespoons powdered sugar,
  plus ½ cup for dredging
¼ teaspoon salt
½ cup (1 stick) margarine,
  chilled

½ cup finely chopped
  hazelnuts
1 teaspoon vanilla
  extract
¼ cup cold water

Using an electric mixer at medium speed, beat flour, 2 tablespoons powdered sugar, salt, and margarine to form a coarse crumb. Add hazelnuts, vanilla, and water and mix at medium speed until the dough pulls together.

Turn the dough out onto a lightly floured work surface and knead a few times to form a smooth ball. Cover and refrigerate for 2 hours to overnight. Return the dough to room temperature.

Divide the dough into 36 equal portions of 1 tablespoon each (level no. 60 dipper). Shape each portion into a roll about 4 inches long with tapered ends. Form the rolls into crescents and place them on cookie sheets that have been sprayed with cooking spray or lined with aluminum foil.

Bake at 350°F for 12 to 15 minutes, or until lightly browned on the bottoms. Dredge the warm crescents in the ½ cup powdered sugar and place on wire racks to cool to room temperature. Store crescents in an airtight container or freeze until needed.

Note: Other kinds of chopped nuts may be used instead of the hazelnuts with very little change in the nutritive values.

Yield: 36 cookies
Food exchanges per cookie: 1 starch; or ½ carbohydrate choice
Sugar per cookie: 0.5 teaspoon or 2 grams
Low-cholesterol diets: Recipe is suitable as written.
Low-sodium diets: Omit salt and use salt-free margarine.
Nutritive values per cookie:

Calories: 60	FAT: 3 g
CHO: 7 g	Na: 45 mg
PRO: 1 g	Cholesterol: 0

CHAPTER 7

$\mathscr{B}$ars

BARS ARE HARD to classify. They are generally baked like a cake and served like a cookie. Occasionally, they are served with ice cream or whipped topping and then again they are served with fruit or on a platter of cookies so they don't really fit into any other category than bars.

You need to remember all of the information regarding baking both cakes and cookies when you are making them but there are some additional guidelines that are meant specially for bars:

1. It is important to use the correct size pan for bars. They are generally baked in an 11 × 15-inch jelly roll pan or a 9 × 13-inch cake pan but sometimes I bake them in a 12 × 18-inch sheet pan, which is generally used for institutional service. If you want to use the larger pan, you need to double the amount of dough used for a 9 × 13-inch cake pan, or use 1⅓ times the amount of batter for an 11 × 15-inch jelly roll pan to fill the 12 × 18-inch sheet pan. If you bake bars in a pan that is too large, they will be too thin, dry, and hard, and if you bake them in a pan that is too small, they may run over the sides of the pan or they will be too soft, more like a cake.

2. Most bars should be cut as soon as they reach room temperature unless the recipe states otherwise.

3. The bars should be cut as directed in the recipe. If you cut them larger or smaller, you will change the food exchanges or carbohydrate grams or choices. If you think the bar is too small and want to cut them twice as large, double the food exchanges or carbohydrate grams or

choices; or if you want dainty bars for a cookie platter, cut them half as large and cut the food exchanges or carbohydrate grams or choices in half also.

4. Store bars in their pans, covered with plastic, aluminum foil, or a plastic cover, until serving time. Most of them freeze well and they can be frozen, tightly covered, in the pan or cut and then frozen in a plastic bag. Most of the bars can be frozen but they should be thawed, still covered, in the refrigerator and then brought to room temperature just before they are served.

Bars are easier to make than cookies, so I make them frequently for potluck dinners, for serving at school or church, or to have on hand when I need them.

When I take them somewhere I label them "Diabetic: 1 starch and 1 fat exchanges or 1 carbohydrate choice" and I never have any left because so many people have diabetes or are on a carbohydrate-controlled diet and they are happy to have them also. I also like to have something available that I know I can eat without worrying about it. They are easy to make, handy, and I enjoy them . . . and hope you will also.

Applesauce Bars

2 cups all-purpose flour
1/3 cup sugar
Dry sugar substitute equal to
  3/4 cup sugar
1 teaspoon cinnamon
1/2 teaspoon nutmeg
1/4 teaspoon cloves

1 1/2 cups hot unsweetened
  applesauce
2 teaspoons baking
  soda
1/3 cup vegetable oil
1/4 cup chopped walnuts
1/4 cup raisins

Place flour, sugar, dry sugar substitute, cinnamon, nutmeg, and cloves in a mixer bowl and mix at low speed to blend well. Combine hot applesauce and baking soda (don't try to be modern and use cold applesauce and mix the baking soda with the flour; it doesn't work as well that way), and add, along with oil, walnuts, and raisins, to flour mixture. Mix at medium speed until flour is moistened and batter is creamy. Spread batter evenly in a 9 × 13-inch cake pan that has been sprayed with cooking spray or greased well with margarine.

Bake at 375°F for 20 to 25 minutes, or until bars pull away from the sides of the pan and a cake tester comes out clean from the center. Cool on a wire rack. Cut three by six.

Yield: 18 servings
Food exchanges per serving: 1 starch and 1 fat; or 1 carbohydrate
  choice
Sugar per serving: .9 teaspoon or 4 grams
Low-cholesterol diets: Recipe is suitable as written.
Low-sodium diets: Recipe is suitable as written.
Nutritive values per serving:

Calories: 122	FAT: 5 g
CHO: 18 g	Na: 92 mg
PRO: 2 g	Cholesterol: 0

Butterscotch Chip Bars

I'm very fond of chocolate chips, but I also like butterscotch chips and think they should be used more often.

⅔ cup (1⅓ sticks) margarine at room temperature
½ cup packed brown sugar
1 tablespoon Sweet 'n Low dry brown sugar substitute
2 teaspoons caramel or burnt flavoring

1 teaspoon vanilla extract
3 large eggs
3 cups all-purpose flour
1½ teaspoons baking soda
½ teaspoon salt
¾ cup butterscotch chips
⅓ cup water at room temperature

Cream margarine, brown sugar, and dry brown sugar substitute together until light and fluffy. Add flavorings and eggs, and mix at medium speed until creamy again, scraping down the bowl before and after addition. Stir flour, baking soda, salt, and butterscotch chips together to blend well, and add, along with the water, to the creamy mixture. Mix at medium speed until creamy again. Spread batter evenly in an 11 × 15-inch jelly roll pan that has been sprayed with cooking spray or greased with margarine.

Bake at 350°F for 25 to 30 minutes, or until bars are well browned and firm in the center. Remove to a wire rack and cool to room temperature. Cut four by seven.

Yield: 28 servings
Food exchanges per serving: 1 starch and 1 fat; or 1 carbohydrate choice
Sugar per serving: .9 teaspoon or 4 grams
Low-cholesterol diets: Omit eggs. Use ¾ cup egg whites or liquid egg substitute.
Low-sodium diets: Omit salt. Use salt-free margarine.
Nutritive values per serving:

Calories: 133
CHO: 17 g
PRO: 2 g

FAT: 7 g
Na: 142 mg
Cholesterol: 29 mg

Carrot Bars

You can use cooked, pureed carrots or you can buy two 4-ounce cans of baby food pureed carrots. Either one will give you a rich, luscious bar.

3 large eggs
1 cup sugar
1/2 cup vegetable oil
1 cup pureed cooked carrots
1 teaspoon vanilla extract
2 cups all-purpose flour
Dry sugar substitute equal to
   1/4 cup sugar (optional)

2 teaspoons baking
   soda
1/2 teaspoon salt
1 1/2 teaspoons
   cinnamon
1/2 cup raisins
1/2 cup chopped English
   walnuts

Place eggs, sugar, oil, carrots, and vanilla in a mixer bowl and mix at medium speed until creamy. Stir flour, dry sugar substitute (if using), baking soda, salt, cinnamon, raisins, and nuts together to blend well, and add to creamy mixture. Mix at medium speed until creamy again. Spread batter evenly in an 11 x 15-inch jelly roll pan that has been sprayed with cooking spray or greased with margarine.

Bake at 350°F for 25 to 30 minutes, or until bars are firm in the center. Remove to a wire rack and cool to room temperature. Cut four by seven.

Yield: 28 servings
Food exchanges per serving: 1 starch and 1 fat; or 1 carbohydrate
   choice
Sugar per serving: 1.7 teaspoons or 7 grams
Low-cholesterol diets: Omit eggs. Use 3/4 cup egg whites or liquid egg
   substitute.
Low-sodium diets: Omit salt. Use salt-free carrot puree.
Nutritive values per serving:

Calories: 135
CHO: 17 g
PRO: 2 g

FAT: 5 g
Na: 110 mg
Cholesterol: 29 mg

Cappuccino Brownies

Cappuccino fans will enjoy these brownies with a hot cup of freshly brewed coffee.

1 tablespoon instant coffee granules	1/3 cup granulated sugar
1 tablespoon boiling water	2 tablespoons cocoa powder
3/4 cup semisweet chocolate chips	2 large eggs
	1/2 teaspoon vanilla extract
1/4 cup butter or margarine, softened	1/2 cup all-purpose flour
	1/4 teaspoon ground cinnamon
	Powdered sugar

In a small bowl, dissolve coffee in water; set aside. In a microwave-safe bowl or saucepan over low heat, melt chocolate chips. Beat butter or margarine, granulated sugar, and cocoa on medium speed until light. Beat in eggs, melted chocolate, coffee mixture, and vanilla. Combine flour and cinnamon; add to the creamed mixture and mix well. Pour into a greased 8-inch square baking pan.

Bake at 350°F for 20 to 30 minutes, or until a toothpick inserted near the center comes out clean. Dust with powdered sugar. Cool on a wire rack. Cut four by four.

Yield: 16 servings
Food exchanges per serving: 1 starch and 1/2 fat; or 1 carbohydrate choice
Sugar per serving: 2.2 teaspoons or 9 grams
Low-cholesterol diets: Omit eggs. Use 1/2 cup liquid egg substitute.
Low-sodium diets: Recipe is suitable as written.
Nutritive values per serving:

Calories: 100	FAT: 6 g
CHO: 13 g	Na: 40 mg
PRO: 2 g	Cholesterol: 25 mg

Chocolate Bars

This recipe is based on my favorite one for fudge brownies, but with enough of the fat and sugar removed to make it suitable for a carbohydrate-controlled diet. These bars go well with lemonade, coffee, or tea.

2 cups all-purpose flour
1 cup sugar
½ cup unsweetened cocoa powder
1 teaspoon baking soda
Dry sugar substitute equal to ⅓ cup sugar
½ teaspoon cinnamon
½ teaspoon salt
1 cup (2 sticks) margarine at room temperature
2 large eggs
2 teaspoons vanilla extract
½ cup water at room temperature
½ cup semisweet chocolate chips

Place flour, sugar, cocoa, baking soda, dry sugar substitute, cinnamon, and salt in a mixer bowl and mix at low speed to blend well. Add margarine, eggs, vanilla, and water, and mix at medium speed to blend. Spread batter evenly in an 11 × 15-inch jelly roll pan that has been sprayed with cooking spray or greased with margarine.

Bake at 325°F for 20 to 25 minutes, or until bars pull away from the sides of the pan and a cake tester comes out clean from the center. Place on a wire rack and sprinkle chocolate chips evenly over the top of the hot bars. Mark four by eight and cool until chocolate has hardened. Cut into 32 bars.

Yield: 32 servings
Food exchanges per serving: 1 starch and 1 fat; or 1 carbohydrate choice
Sugar per serving: 1.5 teaspoons or 6 grams
Low-cholesterol diets: Omit eggs. Use ½ cup egg whites or liquid egg substitute.
Low-sodium diets: Omit salt. Use salt-free margarine.
Nutritive values per serving:

Calories: 123
CHO: 14 g
PRO: 2 g
FAT: 7 g
Na: 97 mg
Cholesterol: 17 mg

Chocolate Chip Bars

This recipe is based on the regular chocolate chip cookies we all enjoy so much.

½ cup (1 stick) margarine at
    room temperature
¾ cup sugar
Dry brown sugar substitute
    equal to ½ cup brown sugar
1 teaspoon vanilla extract

2 large eggs
2¼ cups all-purpose flour
1 teaspoon baking soda
½ teaspoon salt
½ cup semisweet chocolate
    chips

Cream margarine, sugar, and dry brown sugar substitute together at medium speed until light and fluffy. Add vanilla and eggs, and mix at medium speed for 30 seconds, scraping down the bowl before and after addition. Stir flour, baking soda, and salt together to blend, and add to creamy mixture. Mix at medium speed until creamy again; then add chocolate chips. Spread batter evenly in a 9 × 13-inch cake pan that has been sprayed with cooking spray or greased with margarine.

Bake at 375°F for 25 minutes, or until bars are browned and pull away from the sides of the pan. Remove to a wire rack and cool to room temperature. Cut four by six.

Yield: 24 servings
Food exchanges per serving: 1 starch and 1 fat; or 1 carbohydrate
    choice
Sugar per serving: 1.5 teaspoons or 6 grams
Low-cholesterol diets: Omit eggs. Use ½ cup egg whites or liquid egg
    substitute.
Low-sodium diets: Omit salt. Use salt-free margarine.
Nutritive values per serving:

Calories: 125
CHO: 17 g
PRO: 2 g

FAT: 6 g
Na: 129 mg
Cholesterol: 23 mg

Chocolate Chip Oatmeal Bars

These bars are a favorite of John Franks, of Oelwein, Iowa. The Franks were our next-door neighbors when John was younger. We called him Johnathan then; now he is in high school and wants to be called John, but he still loves chocolate chip cookies and bars.

¾ cup (1½ sticks) margarine at room temperature
½ cup granulated sugar
⅓ cup packed brown sugar
2 large eggs
2 teaspoons vanilla extract
1 cup all-purpose flour

2 cups rolled oats
1 teaspoon baking soda
½ teaspoon salt
½ cup semisweet chocolate chips
½ cup water at room temperature

Cream margarine and sugars together until light and fluffy. Add eggs and vanilla, and mix at medium speed until creamy, scraping down the bowl before and after addition. Stir flour, oats, baking soda, salt, and chocolate chips together lightly to blend. Add, along with water, to creamy mixture, and mix until oats are absorbed. Spread batter evenly in an 11 × 15-inch jelly roll pan that has been sprayed with cooking spray or greased with margarine.

Bake at 350°F for 20 to 25 minutes, or until bars are firm and lightly browned. Place on a wire rack and cool to room temperature. Cut four by seven.

Yield: 28 servings
Food exchanges per serving: 1 starch and 1 fat; or 1 carbohydrate choice
Sugar per serving: 1.4 teaspoons or 6 grams
Low-cholesterol diets: Omit eggs. Use ½ cup egg whites or liquid egg substitute.
Low-sodium diets: Omit salt. Use salt-free margarine.
Nutritive values per serving:

Calories: 126
CHO: 15 g
PRO: 2 g

FAT: 7 g
Na: 131 mg
Cholesterol: 20 mg

Easy Microwave Toffee Bars

The alluring tastes of chocolate and peanut butter come together in these quick-to-make bars. A must-have treat for children and adults of *all* ages.

5½ double 5 × 2½-inch graham crackers
1 cup crushed (6 double 5 × 2½-inch) graham crackers
½ cup granulated sugar
⅓ cup packed brown sugar
⅓ cup margarine or butter
⅓ cup fat-free milk
⅓ cup semisweet chocolate chips
¼ cup chunky peanut butter

Line the bottom of a buttered 12 × 8-inch baking dish with graham crackers; set aside. In a 2-quart casserole, combine all remaining ingredients except chocolate chips and peanut butter. Microwave on high for about 1½ to 2 minutes, stirring after 1 minute, or until mixture comes to a full boil. Mix again and then microwave on high for another 3 to 4 minutes (mixture will be very hot). Watch closely so mixture does not separate or start to burn. Immediately pour mixture evenly over crackers.

In 2-cup glass measuring cup, combine chocolate chips and peanut butter. Microwave on high until chocolate is softened, 45 to 60 seconds. Stir until smooth and melted. Spread evenly over toffee mixture; refrigerate until chocolate is set, at least 1½ hours. Cut into 32 bars; store at room temperature.

Yield: 32 servings
Food exchanges per serving: 1 starch; or 1 carbohydrate choice
Sugar per serving: 1.7 teaspoons or 7 grams
Low-cholesterol diets: Recipe is suitable as written. You may want to use reduced-fat peanut butter to further lower the fat content.
Low-sodium diets: You may want to use salt-free margarine and low-sodium peanut butter.
Nutritive values per serving:

Calories: 70
CHO: 9 g
PRO: 1 g
FAT: 3.5 g
Na: 50 mg
Cholesterol: 0

Ginger Bars

The recipe for these bars came from my friend Vivian Lott, of Volga, Iowa, who makes them frequently for her family. She has four boys at home, and they can eat a pan of these in one after-school session.

½ cup packed brown sugar	½ teaspoon salt
½ cup molasses	1 teaspoon cinnamon
½ cup vegetable shortening	1 teaspoon ginger
2 large eggs	1 cup hot coffee
2½ cups all-purpose flour	3 tablespoons granulated
1 teaspoon baking soda	sugar

Place brown sugar, molasses, and shortening in a mixer bowl and mix at medium speed until creamy. Add eggs and mix at medium speed for 30 seconds, scraping down the bowl before and after addition. Stir flour, baking soda, salt, cinnamon, and ginger together to blend well. Add flour mixture, along with coffee, to creamy mixture. Mix at medium speed until creamy again. Spread batter evenly in an 11 × 15-inch jelly roll pan that has been sprayed with cooking spray or greased with margarine. Sprinkle granulated sugar evenly over batter.

Bake at 350°F for 30 minutes, or until bars pull away from the sides of the pan and a cake tester comes out clean from the center. Remove to a wire rack and cool to room temperature. Cut five by six.

Yield: 30 servings
Food exchanges per serving: 1 starch and 1 fat; or 1 carbohydrate choice
Sugar per serving: 1.9 teaspoons or 8 grams
Low-cholesterol diets: Omit eggs. Use ½ cup egg whites or liquid egg substitute.
Low-sodium diets: Omit salt.
Nutritive values per serving:

Calories: 103	FAT: 4 g
CHO: 16 g	Na: 74 mg
PRO: 1 g	Cholesterol: 18 mg

Oatmeal Squares

⅓ cup sugar
Dry brown sugar substitute
   equal to ½ cup brown sugar
¼ cup (½ stick) margarine at
   room temperature
1 teaspoon vanilla extract
1 large egg

2 tablespoons water
¾ cup all-purpose flour
1 teaspoon baking
   powder
1½ cups old-fashioned
   rolled oats
¼ cup chopped nuts

Beat sugar, sugar substitute, margarine, and vanilla at medium speed until light and fluffy. Add egg and water and beat until blended. Stir flour and baking powder together and add to creamy mixture. Mix well. Add oats and nuts and mix. Spread evenly in a lightly greased 9-inch square pan.

Bake at 350°F for 25 to 30 minutes, or until a toothpick comes out clean. Cool for 30 minutes. Cut four by four. Cool an additional 15 minutes before serving.

Yield: 16 servings
Food exchanges per serving: 1 starch and 1 fat; or 1 carbohydrate
   choice
Sugar per serving: 1 teaspoon or 4 grams
Low-cholesterol diets: Omit egg. Use ¼ cup egg whites or liquid egg
   substitute.
Low-sodium diets: Use low-sodium baking powder.
Nutritive values per serving:

Calories: 140
CHO: 20 g
PRO: 3 g

FAT: 8 g
Na: 100 mg
Cholesterol: 15 mg

Pioneer Bars

I call these Pioneer Bars because they are based on a recipe from my grandmother, who learned the recipe from her mother. It includes cinnamon, which was available and popular in the days of the early settlers on the Iowa plains.

½ cup raisins
½ cup granulated sugar
1½ cups water
½ cup (1 stick) margarine
1½ teaspoons cinnamon
3 cups all-purpose flour
1½ teaspoons baking soda

½ teaspoon salt
Dry sugar substitute equal to ¼ cup sugar (optional)
2 large eggs
½ cup chopped walnuts
2 tablespoons powdered sugar

Place raisins, granulated sugar, water, margarine, and cinnamon in a pan. Stir, over low heat, to dissolve the sugar; simmer for 2 minutes. Remove pan from heat and cool mixture to room temperature.

Place flour, baking soda, salt, and dry sugar substitute (if using) in a mixer bowl and mix at low speed to blend well. Add cooled raisin mixture, eggs, and walnuts, and mix at medium speed until creamy. Spread batter evenly in an 11 × 15-inch jelly roll pan that has been sprayed with cooking spray or greased with margarine.

Bake at 350°F for 25 to 30 minutes, or until the center of bars springs back when touched. Sprinkle with powdered sugar and cool to room temperature. Cut four by eight.

Yield: 32 servings
Food exchanges per serving: 1 starch and 1 fat; or 1 carbohydrate choice
Sugar per serving: 0.8 teaspoon or 3 grams
Low-cholesterol diets: Omit eggs. Use ½ cup egg whites or liquid egg substitute.
Low-sodium diets: Omit salt. Use salt-free margarine.
Nutritive values per serving:

Calories: 106
CHO: 15 g
PRO: 2 g

FAT: 5 g
Na: 77 mg
Cholesterol: 16 mg

Pumpkin Bars

Here is another recipe from Vivian Lott. They are spicy and just right for an after-school snack, and her sons love them.

3 large eggs	2 cups all-purpose flour
2/3 cup sugar	2 teaspoons cinnamon
Dry brown sugar substitute equal to 1/2 cup brown sugar	2 teaspoons baking powder
1/2 cup vegetable oil	1 teaspoon baking soda
16-ounce can solid pack pumpkin	1/2 teaspoon salt

Place eggs, sugar, dry brown sugar substitute, oil, and pumpkin in a mixer bowl and mix at medium speed until smooth. Stir flour, cinnamon, baking powder, baking soda, and salt together to blend, and add to creamy mixture. Mix at medium speed until creamy again. Spread batter evenly in an 11 × 15-inch jelly roll pan that has been sprayed with cooking spray or greased with margarine.

Bake at 350°F for 25 minutes, or until a cake tester comes out clean from the center of the pan. Remove to a wire rack and cool to room temperature. Cut four by six.

Note: These are good served with fruit or pudding, or topped with a couple of tablespoons of whipped diabetic topping. There will be no change in exchanges if whipped diabetic topping is used.

Yield: 24 servings
Food exchanges per serving: 1 starch and 1 fat; or 1 carbohydrate choice
Sugar per serving: 1.3 teaspoons or 5 grams
Low-cholesterol diets: Omit eggs. Use 3/4 cup egg whites or liquid egg substitute.
Low-sodium diets: Omit salt. Use low-sodium baking powder.
Nutritive values per serving:

Calories: 117	FAT: 5 g
CHO: 15 g	Na: 116 mg
PRO: 2 g	Cholesterol: 34 mg

Raspberry-Almond Bars

My family enjoys the delicate combination of raspberries and almonds in these scrumptious bars.

⅓ cup butter or margarine
¾ cup vanilla or white
   chocolate chips
2 large eggs
⅓ cup sugar
1 teaspoon almond extract

1 cup all-purpose flour
¼ teaspoon salt
½ cup all-fruit, low-sugar
   seedless raspberry
   preserves
¼ cup sliced almonds

In a saucepan, melt butter. Remove from the heat; add half of the chips (do not stir). Set aside.

Beat eggs until foamy; gradually beat in sugar. Stir in butter mixture and almond extract. Combine flour and salt; add to egg mixture and mix just until combined. Spread half of the batter into a greased 9-inch square baking pan.

Bake at 325°F for 15 to 20 minutes, or until golden brown.

In a small saucepan over low heat, melt preserves; spread over warm crust. Stir remaining chips into the remaining batter; drop by teaspoonfuls over the preserves layer. Sprinkle with almonds. Bake 30 to 35 minutes longer, or until a toothpick inserted near the center comes out clean. Cool on a wire rack. Cut six by four.

Yield: 24 servings
Food exchanges per serving: 1 starch and ½ fat; or 1 carbohydrate
   choice
Sugar per serving: 2 teaspoons or 8 grams
Low-cholesterol diets: Omit eggs. Use ½ cup egg whites or liquid egg
   substitute.
Low-sodium diets: Omit salt.
Nutritive values per serving:

Calories: 105
CHO: 13 g
PRO: 2 g

FAT: 5 g
Na: 72 mg
Cholesterol: 18 mg

Rice Krispies Treats

Many people are already familiar with this recipe but I thought you might like to have it, along with its nutritive values, so you could fit it more easily into your meal plan.

¼ cup (½ stick) margarine
10-ounce package (about 40)
    large marshmallows or 4 cups
    miniature marshmallows

6 cups Kellogg's Rice Krispies

Melt margarine in a large saucepan over low heat. Add marshmallows and stir until completely melted. Remove from heat. Add Rice Krispies and stir until coated. With a spatula or wax paper that has been greased with margarine, press mixture evenly into a 9 × 13-inch cake pan that has been well greased with margarine. Cool to room temperature. Cut five by six into 30 bars.

Directions for microwave: Microwave margarine and marshmallows on full power in a large glass mixing bowl for 2 minutes. Stir to combine. Microwave for another 1½ to 2 minutes. Stir until smooth. Add cereal and stir until well coated. Press, cool, and cut as directed in basic recipe.

Yield: 30 servings
Food exchanges per serving: ½ starch; or ½ carbohydrate choice
Sugar per serving: 0.5 teaspoon or 2 grams
Low-cholesterol diets: Recipe is suitable as written.
Low-sodium diets: Use salt-free margarine.
Nutritive values per serving:

Calories: 66	FAT: 1 g
CHO: 8 g	Na: 70 mg
PRO: 0	Cholesterol: 0

Strawberry-Almond Chocolate Bars

I like to take these bars to potlucks, community functions, and family gatherings. There are never any left to take back home.

Crumb Mixture

2 cups all-purpose flour
1/3 cup sugar

2/3 cup butter or margarine at room temperature

Filling

1 cup low-sugar strawberry preserves
2 1/2-ounce package (2/3 cup) sliced almonds

1/2 teaspoon almond extract

Glaze

1/3 cup milk or semisweet chocolate chips
1 tablespoon butter

1/4 cup powdered sugar
2 tablespoons fat-free milk
1/2 teaspoon vanilla extract

In large mixer bowl combine all crust mixture ingredients. Beat at low speed, scraping bowl often, until well mixed, 2 to 3 minutes. Press crust mixture on bottom of 9 × 13-inch baking pan. Bake at 350°F for 20 to 25 minutes, or until edges are lightly browned.

In same mixer bowl stir together all filling ingredients. Spread filling over hot crust.

Melt chocolate chips and butter in a small saucepan over low heat, stirring occasionally, until smooth, 2 to 3 minutes. Stir in all remaining glaze ingredients. Drizzle warm glaze over bars. If glaze is too thick, stir in a little extra milk. Cool completely. Cut four by nine.

Yield: 36 servings
Food exchanges per serving: 1 starch and 1 fat; or 1 carbohydrate choice
Sugar per serving: 1.4 teaspoons or 6 grams
Low-cholesterol diets: Recipe is suitable as written. May want to use margarine.
Low-sodium diets: Recipe is suitable as written. May want to use salt-free margarine.
Nutritive values per serving:

Calories: 100	FAT: 5 g
CHO: 12 g	Na: 40 mg
PRO: 1 g	Cholesterol: 5 mg

Strawberry Pizza

Cheesecake and strawberry lovers will be delighted with this fruity treat.

5 tablespoons butter or
  margarine, softened
1/4 cup sugar
Dry sugar substitute equal to 4
  teaspoons sugar
1 large egg

1/2 teaspoon vanilla extract
1/4 teaspoon almond
  extract
1 1/4 cups all-purpose flour
1/2 teaspoon baking powder
1/2 teaspoon salt

Filling

8 ounces (1 cup) reduced-fat
  cream cheese at room
  temperature
1/3 cup powdered sugar

2 cups sliced strawberries
2 cups crushed strawberries
0.6-ounce package sugar-free
  strawberry gelatin

Beat butter, sugar, and dry sugar substitute at medium speed for 2 minutes. Beat in egg and extracts. Combine flour, baking powder, and salt; gradually add to creamy mixture and mix well. Cover and refrigerate for 1 hour.

On a floured surface, roll dough into a 13-inch circle. Transfer to an ungreased 12-inch pizza pan. Build up edges slightly.

Bake at 350°F for 18 to 22 minutes, or until lightly browned. Cool completely.

For filling: Beat cream cheese and powdered sugar until smooth. Spread over crust. Arrange sliced strawberries on top.

In a saucepan bring crushed strawberries to a boil. Cook, stirring, for 2 minutes. Remove from heat. Add strawberry gelatin and mix until it is completely dissolved. Cool slightly until gelatin starts to set. Spoon over strawberries. Refrigerate until serving. Cut into 14 equal slices.

Yield: 14 servings
Food exchanges per serving: 1 starch, 1 fruit, and 1 fat; or 1
  carbohydrate choice
Sugar per serving: 2.4 teaspoons or 10 grams
Low-cholesterol diets: Omit egg. Use 1/4 cup liquid egg substitute.
  May use fat-free cream cheese as desired in place of reduced-fat
  cream cheese.
Low-sodium diets: Omit salt. Use salt-free margarine and low-sodium
  baking powder.
Nutritive values per serving:

Calories: 160   FAT: 7 g
CHO: 20 g   Na: 200 mg
PRO: 4 g   Cholesterol: 25 mg

Zucchini Bars

Summer zucchini squash finds its way from the vegetable garden to the dessert course in these easy-to-make bars. These delicious, moist bars are packed with both great taste and nutrition. These bars freeze well if you like to bake ahead for unexpected guests.

1¼ cups sugar
4 large eggs
½ cup vegetable oil
½ cup unsweetened applesauce
2 cups grated zucchini

¼ teaspoon salt
2¼ cups all-purpose flour
1 teaspoon cinnamon
2 teaspoons baking powder
2 teaspoons baking soda

Beat sugar, eggs, and oil at medium speed until light. Add applesauce and mix until smooth. Add remaining ingredients and mix until blended. Pour batter into a large (12 × 17-inch) cookie sheet that has been sprayed with cooking spray.

Bake at 350°F for 30 to 35 minutes or until top springs back when lightly pressed. Cut five by eight.

Yield: 40 servings (unfrosted bars)
Food exchanges per serving: 1 starch; or 1 carbohydrate choice
Sugar per serving: 1.7 teaspoons or 7 grams
Low-cholesterol diets: Omit eggs. Use 1 cup egg whites or liquid egg substitute.
Low-sodium diets: Omit salt. Use low-sodium baking powder.
Nutritive values per bar:

Calories: 84
CHO: 12 g
PRO: 1 g

FAT: 3 g
Na: 109 mg
Cholesterol: 21 mg

Cream Cheese Frosting

¾ cup (6 ounces) reduced-fat cream cheese
¼ cup margarine

1 teaspoon vanilla extract
2 cups powdered sugar
Fat-free milk as needed

Allow cream cheese and margarine to soften at room temperature for about 1 hour. Beat the margarine and cream cheese until smooth. Add vanilla and mix well. Add powdered sugar, 1 cup at a time, mixing well after each addition. Add small amounts of milk, 1 teaspoon at a time, until frosting reaches desired consistency. Spread evenly over cooled bars. Enough frosting for 12 × 17-inch pan.

Yield: 40 servings (frosted bars)

Food exchanges per serving: 1 starch and 1 fat; or 1 carbohydrate choice

Sugar per serving: 2.9 teaspoons or 12 grams

Nutritive values per frosted bar:

Calories: 127	FAT: 5 g
CHO: 17 g	Na: 140 mg
PRO: 1.5 g	Cholesterol: 23 mg

CHAPTER 8

Pies and Pastries

PIES AND PASTRIES are special treats reserved for special occasions, so you want them to be as close to perfect as possible when you serve them. If you have ever had difficulty preparing pies and pastries, following these simple precautions may help:

1. Use only high-quality, fresh ingredients, and have everything you will need ready for use when you start preparing the recipe. All ingredients are presumed to be at room temperature unless specified differently in the recipe; when it is particularly important they be at room temperature, it is stated in the recipe. Use clean utensils, and use the ones indicated in the recipe. All measures are level, and standard measuring spoons and cups should be used for good results.

2. Avoid making substitutions in the recipe unless you are sure of the substitution ratio and the effect of the substitute item on the nutritive and food exchange or carbohydrate values.

3. Check your oven occasionally for accuracy. The wrong oven temperature can wreck a recipe as fast as the wrong ingredients. Use the pan size indicated in the recipe. Filling meant for a 10-inch pie will overwhelm an 8-inch crust, and filling meant for an 8-inch pie will be woefully inadequate in a 10-inch crust.

4. Dough for piecrust may be mixed in a mixer or by hand. Do not overmix the dough. Overmixing will cause a crust to be tough and shrink while it is baking. Dough should be eased gently into the pie pan, as it will shrink if it is stretched too much.

5. Piecrust dough should be refrigerated when not being used. If the dough becomes too warm, the fat will melt and the baked crust will not be flaky.

6. Baking temperatures for crusts are very important. A crust baked at too low a temperature will be tough; one baked at too high a temperature will be browned on the outside and raw in the center.

7. When using any of the piecrusts to fashion your own pie recipe, add the nutritive values for the crust to those of the filling for the total values per serving.

Remember, you may have pie if you work it into your meal plan. You'll probably have to give up something else, but if pie is your idea of a gastronomical treat, you may enjoy it as long as you plan for it.

Graham Cracker Piecrust

This crust can be prepared ahead of time and frozen. That makes it very handy when you need a dessert for an unexpected guest or for a last-minute potluck dinner.

8 graham crackers (2½-inch squares)
½ teaspoon Sweet 'n Low brown sugar substitute

½ teaspoon cinnamon
2 tablespoons sugar
3 tablespoons margarine

Crush graham crackers (I put them in a plastic bag and crush them with a rolling pin). Add brown sugar substitute, cinnamon, and sugar, and blend well. Melt margarine in a 9-inch pie pan. Add crumb mixture to melted margarine, and mix well with fingers. Press crumb mixture evenly over the bottom and sides of the pie pan.

Bake at 350°F for 6 minutes. Cool to room temperature. Fill and cut pie into 6 or 8 equal slices.

Yield: 6 servings (1 piecrust)
Food exchanges per serving: ⅔ starch and 1 fat; or 1 carbohydrate choice
Sugar per serving: 1 teaspoon or 4 grams
Low-cholesterol diets: Recipe is suitable as written.
Low-sodium diets: Recipe is suitable as written.
Nutritive values per serving:

Calories: 104
CHO: 11 g
PRO: 1 g

FAT: 7 g
Na: 130 mg
Cholesterol: 0

Yield: 8 servings (1 piecrust)
Food exchanges per serving: ½ starch and 1 fat; or 1 carbohydrate choice
Sugar per serving: 1 teaspoon or 4 grams
Low-cholesterol diets: Recipe is suitable as written.
Low-sodium diets: Recipe is suitable as written.
Nutritive values per serving:

Calories: 78
CHO: 8 g
PRO: 1 g

FAT: 5 g
Na: 98 mg
Cholesterol: 0

Hot-Water Piecrust

This crust is more tender than flaky. It is the first crust I learned to make as a teenager, and I'm still making it.

½ cup vegetable shortening	½ teaspoon baking
½ cup boiling water	powder
1½ cups all-purpose flour	½ teaspoon salt

Combine shortening and water, and stir with a fork until creamy and shortening is dissolved. Set aside and cool to room temperature.

Place flour, baking powder, and salt in a bowl and stir to blend well. Add cooled shortening mixture to flour mixture; stir with a fork to blend well. (Add up to 2 tablespoons lukewarm water, if necessary, for a smooth dough, depending on the kind of flour you are using.) Form dough into a ball, cover, and refrigerate from 3 hours to overnight.

Return dough to room temperature before you use it. Divide into 2 equal portions, form into balls, and roll each ball out on a lightly floured board to form a circle 10 inches in diameter. Fit each circle into a 9-inch pie pan that has been sprayed with cooking spray or greased lightly with margarine. If the crust is to be filled before baking, follow the specific pie recipe. If the crust is to be filled after baking, prick the bottom of the crust several times with a fork and bake at 425°F for 12 to 15 minutes, or until crust is lightly browned; then cool and fill. Cut filled pie into 8 equal slices. Makes 2 piecrusts.

Note: Each crust is considered to have been cut into 8 equal servings for the nutritive information.

Yield: 16 servings (2 piecrusts, 8 servings each)
Food exchanges per serving: ⅔ starch and 1 fat; or 1 carbohydrate choice
Sugar per serving: None
Low-cholesterol diets: Recipe is suitable as written.
Low-sodium diets: Omit salt.
Nutritive values per serving:

Calories: 99	FAT: 7 g
CHO: 9 g	Na: 77 mg
PRO: 1 g	Cholesterol: 0

Margarine Piecrust

This crust is crisp and tasty even though it doesn't have as much margarine as I used to use before I developed diabetes.

1 cup all-purpose flour	¼ cup (½ stick) margarine from the refrigerator
¼ teaspoon salt	About ⅓ cup very cold water

Stir flour and salt together to blend. Add margarine and, using a pastry knife, cut the margarine into small pieces to form a coarse crumb. Add water and mix with a fork to form a ball. Knead lightly two or three times on a lightly floured board and roll out to form a single round crust about 9 or 10 inches in diameter. (You may also refrigerate dough for 2 hours to overnight, then bring back to room temperature and roll out as instructed.)

Spray an 8- or 9-inch pie pan with cooking spray or grease lightly with margarine, and ease the crust evenly into the pan. If the crust is to be baked and then filled, prick the bottom with a fork several times and bake at 425° to 450°F for about 15 minutes, or until crust is lightly browned. Cool and fill. If the crust is to be filled and then baked, bake according to directions. Cut the crust into 8 equal pieces.

Note: Filling should be lukewarm or cold when placed in the unbaked crust; a hot filling will ruin the crust. When baking the crust to be filled later, place an empty pie tin over the crust for the first 10 minutes in the oven.

Yield: 8 servings (1 piecrust)
Food exchanges per serving: ⅓ starch and 1 fat; or 1 carbohydrate choice
Sugar per serving: None
Low-cholesterol diets: Recipe is suitable as written.
Low-sodium diets: Omit salt. Use salt-free margarine.
Nutritive values per serving:

Calories: 108	FAT: 6 g
CHO: 12 g	Na: 137 mg
PRO: 2 g	Cholesterol: 0

Shortening Piecrust

1 cup all-purpose flour   1/3 cup vegetable shortening
1/2 teaspoon salt   1/4 cup very cold water

Mix flour and salt in a bowl. With a pastry blender/cutter cut in the vegetable shortening until mixture is crumbly. Stir in cold water and work dough gently with your hands just until it forms a ball. Do not overwork or the piecrust will be tough.

Roll dough out on a floured surface. Place in 9-inch pie pan. Trim and flute edges. For a prebaked crust, prick holes in the crust with a fork and bake at 425°F for 10 to 12 minutes, or until light golden brown.

Yield: 8 servings
Food exchanges per serving: 1 starch and 1 fat; or 1 carbohydrate choice
Sugar per serving: None
Low-cholesterol diets: Recipe is suitable as written.
Low-sodium diets: Omit salt.
Nutritive values per serving:

Calories: 117	FAT: 7 g
CHO: 12 g	Na: 117 mg
PRO: 2 g	Cholesterol: 0

Nutritive values for whole crust:

Calories: 936	FAT: 55 g
CHO: 95 g	Na: 936 mg
PRO: 13 g	Cholesterol: 0

Apple Flan

Apple Flan is similar to a custard pie, only it is made with fruit. If you enjoy the taste of apple pie, but do not have time to peel apples, this is a delicious and simple dessert solution.

9-inch Shortening Piecrust
  (page 157)
1 tablespoon butter, melted
1 cup unsweetened
  applesauce
2½ tablespoons lemon juice
⅓ cup sugar
Dry sugar substitute equal to
  ⅓ cup sugar

4 eggs
¼ teaspoon vanilla extract
½ teaspoon apple pie spice
⅛ teaspoon salt
Cinnamon
Whipped cream or light
  whipped topping
Fresh apple slices
Mint sprigs

Prepare crust and partially bake; set aside.

Mix together butter, applesauce, lemon juice, sugar, sugar substitute, eggs, vanilla, apple pie spice, and salt until well blended. Pour apple mixture into pie shell.

Bake at 325°F for about 1 hour, or until filling is set and top is golden brown. A knife inserted into the center of the pie will come out clean when the filling is done.

Sprinkle top of the flan with cinnamon. Chill until completely cooled. Garnish each serving with a dollop of whipped cream or light topping, apple slices, and mint leaves. Cut into 8 or 10 equal slices.

Yield: 8 servings
Food exchanges per serving: 1½ starch, 1 fruit, and 2 fat; or 2 carbohydrate choices
Sugar per serving: 3.4 teaspoons or 14 grams
Low-cholesterol diets: Omit eggs. Use 1 cup liquid egg substitute. Use margarine instead of butter.
Low-sodium diets: Omit salt. Use unsalted butter. Omit salt in piecrust.
Nutritive values per serving:

Calories: 255	FAT: 14 g
CHO: 27 g	Na: 225 mg
PRO: 5 g	Cholesterol: 124 mg

Yield: 10 servings

Food exchanges per serving: 1 starch, ½ fruit, and 2 fat; or
1½ carbohydrate choices

Sugar per serving: 2.6 teaspoons or 11 grams

Low-cholesterol diets: Omit eggs. Use 1 cup liquid egg substitute. Use
margarine instead of butter.

Low-sodium diets: Omit salt. Use unsalted butter. Omit salt in piecrust.

Nutritive values per serving:

Calories: 205	**FAT: 12 g**
CHO: 21 g	**Na: 180 mg**
PRO: 4 g	**Cholesterol: 100 mg**

Impossible Pumpkin Pie

I owe the credit for this recipe to my friend Mary Boineau, of Tampa, Florida. We were talking about impossible pies one evening, and she told me that she always adds ½ cup Bisquick to her pumpkin pie recipe and it comes out just fine. I tried her method, and the pie really was good that way.

16-ounce can solid pack pumpkin

2 large eggs

12-ounce can evaporated fat-free milk

Dry brown sugar substitute equal to ½ cup brown sugar

½ cup buttermilk biscuit mix

2 to 3 teaspoons pumpkin pie spice

½ teaspoon salt

Combine all ingredients in a mixer bowl and mix at medium speed until smooth. Pour into a 9-inch pie pan that has been sprayed with cooking spray or greased with margarine.

Bake at 375°F for about 45 minutes, or until a knife comes out clean from the center of the pie. Remove to a wire rack. Cut pie into 8 equal slices. Serve warm or at room temperature.

Note: If you use a metal or foil pie pan (rather than glass or ceramic), place the pan on a preheated cookie sheet in the center of the oven.

Yield: 8 servings
Food exchanges per serving: 1 starch and ½ fat; or 1 carbohydrate choice
Sugar per serving: None
Low-cholesterol diets: Omit eggs. Use ½ cup egg whites or liquid egg substitute.
Low-sodium diets: Omit salt.
Nutritive values per serving:

Calories: 117
CHO: 17 g
PRO: 7 g

FAT: 3 g
Na: 318 mg
Cholesterol: 71 mg

Creamy Banana Dream Pie

If you enjoy banana cream pie, then this lower-fat, lower-sugar version will be sure to delight you. We've trimmed the carbohydrates but kept the taste of a treasured, traditional favorite. Garnish with whipped topping if desired.

9-inch Shortening Piecrust
(page 157)
2 bananas, thinly sliced
Lemon or orange juice
12-ounce can evaporated fat-
free milk, chilled

1-ounce package reduced-
calorie, sugar-free instant
banana cream pudding and
pie filling mix
½ cup plain nonfat yogurt
1 teaspoon vanilla extract

Prepare crust and bake. Set aside.

Dip banana slices in lemon or orange juice to prevent them from turning brown. Drain and set aside.

Beat the evaporated milk, pudding mix, yogurt, and vanilla until mixture starts to thicken. Pour half of pudding mixture into the cooled crust. Arrange banana slices over pudding mixture and top with remaining pudding mixture. Cover and refrigerate until firm. Cut into 8 or 10 equal slices.

Yield: 8 servings
Food exchanges per serving: 1 starch, 1 fruit, and ½ fat; or 2
    carbohydrate choices
Sugar per serving: 3 teaspoons or 13 grams
Low-cholesterol diets: Recipe is suitable as written.
Low-sodium diets: Omit salt in piecrust. Use your own discretion for
    inclusion in your diet.
Nutritive values per serving:

Calories: 166   FAT: 5 g
CHO: 28 g   Na: 310 mg
PRO: 5 g   Cholesterol: 10 mg

Yield: 10 servings
Food exchanges per serving: 1 starch, ½ fruit, and ½ fat; or 1½
    carbohydrate choices
Sugar per serving: 2.4 teaspoons or 10 grams
Low-cholesterol diets: Recipe is suitable as written.
Low-sodium diets: Omit salt in piecrust. Use your own discretion for
    inclusion in your diet.
Nutritive values per serving:

Calories: 133   FAT: 4 g
CHO: 22 g   Na: 248 mg
PRO: 4 g   Cholesterol: 8 mg

Banana Cream Pie

I'm sure many of you have made this pie but I thought it would be a good idea to include it as a basic recipe so you will know the nutritive values when you want to make it.

9-inch Graham Cracker Piecrust (page 154)
2 (1-ounce) packages sugar-free instant vanilla pudding mix
3½ cups fat-free milk

2 medium bananas
About 1-ounce package sugar-free whipped topping mix or 2 cups light whipped topping

Prepare crust and bake. Set aside.

Combine pudding mix and milk, and beat together until smooth. Slice bananas and stir into pudding mixture. Pour into piecrust and refrigerate until firm. If desired, prepare whipped topping according to package directions or use whipped topping and spread evenly over filling. (If you do not use the topping, subtract 10 calories and 19 mg sodium from the nutritive values listed below.) Refrigerate until served. Cut pie into 8 equal slices.

Yield: 8 servings
Food exchanges per serving: 1 starch, ⅔ fruit, and 1 fat; or 2 carbohydrate choices
Sugar per serving: None
Low-cholesterol diets: Recipe is suitable as written.
Low-sodium diets: Recipe is suitable at your discretion. Use salt-free margarine in crust.
Nutritive values per serving:

Calories: 184
CHO: 26 g
PRO: 5 g

FAT: 5 g
Na: 491 mg
Cholesterol: 0 mg

Variations: Vanilla Pudding Pie: Omit bananas.

Chocolate Fudge Pudding Pie: Omit bananas. Use 2 (1-ounce) packages sugar-free instant chocolate fudge pudding mix instead of vanilla.

Butterscotch Pudding Pie: Omit bananas. Use 2 (1-ounce) packages sugar-free instant butterscotch pudding mix instead of vanilla.

Yield: 8 servings

Food exchanges per serving: 1 starch, ⅓ skim milk, and 1 fat; or 1 carbohydrate choice

Sugar per serving: None

Low-cholesterol diets: Recipes are suitable as written.

Low-sodium diets: Recipes are suitable at your discretion. Use salt-free margarine in crust.

Nutritive values per serving:

Calories: 158	FAT: 5 g
CHO: 19 g	Na: 491 mg
PRO: 5 g	Cholesterol: 0 mg

Cherry Pie

9-inch Margarine Piecrust
(page 156)
2 (16-ounce) cans water-packed
red tart cherries
Dry sugar substitute equal to 1
cup sugar
3 tablespoons quick-cooking
tapioca

¼ cup sugar
3 drops red food coloring
¼ teaspoon almond
flavoring
About 1-ounce package
sugar-free whipped topping
mix or 2 cups light whipped
topping

Prepare crust and bake. Set aside.

Combine cherries, including juice, and half of the dry sugar substitute (equal to ½ cup sugar). Mix lightly and let stand, covered, at room temperature for 1 to 2 hours. Drain cherries well, reserving liquid, and set cherries aside. Combine liquid from cherries, tapioca, and sugar, and let stand at room temperature for 15 minutes. Cook over medium heat, stirring constantly, until mixture is thickened and clearer. Remove from heat. Add coloring, flavoring, and remaining dry sugar substitute; mix lightly. Cool to room temperature.

Spread filling evenly in piecrust and refrigerate for at least 30 minutes. Prepare whipped topping according to package directions or use whipped topping and spread evenly over filling. Cut pie into 8 equal slices.

Yield: 8 servings
Food exchanges per serving: 1 starch, 1 fruit, and 1 fat; or 2
carbohydrate choices
Sugar per serving: 1.5 teaspoons or 6 grams
Low-cholesterol diets: Recipe is suitable as written.
Low-sodium diets: In crust, omit salt and use salt-free margarine.
Nutritive values per serving:

Calories: 186   FAT: 6 g
CHO: 30 g   Na: 163 mg
PRO: 3 g   Cholesterol: 0

Chocolate Rum Pie

Other flavorings, such as peppermint, cherry, or orange, may be used in this filling.

9-inch Graham Cracker Piecrust (page 154)
1 envelope Knox gelatin
1/4 cup water at room temperature
1 1/4 cups boiling water
1/2 cup semisweet chocolate chips

1/3 cup instant nonfat dry milk
Dry sugar substitute equal to 1/2 cup sugar
1/4 teaspoon salt
1 teaspoon rum flavoring
About 1-ounce package sugar-free whipped topping mix or 2 cups light whipped topping

Prepare crust and bake. Set aside.

Place gelatin in mixer bowl, add room temperature water, and let stand for 2 to 3 minutes. Add boiling water and stir with whip to dissolve gelatin. Add chocolate chips and continue to stir until chocolate chips are dissolved. Add dry milk, dry sugar substitute, salt, and flavoring, and mix to blend; refrigerate until syrupy.

Beat at high speed for 3 to 5 minutes and pour into piecrust. Refrigerate until firm. Meanwhile prepare whipped topping according to package directions or use whipped topping and spread evenly over filling. After topping is firm, cut pie into 8 equal slices.

Yield: 8 servings
Food exchanges per serving: 2 starch and 3 fat; or 2 carbohydrate choices
Sugar per serving: 1 teaspoon or 4 grams
Low-cholesterol diets: Use fat-free topping.
Low-sodium diets: Omit salt. Use salt-free margarine in crust.
Nutritive values per serving:

Calories: 204
CHO: 28 g
PRO: 4 g

FAT: 14 g
Na: 153 mg
Cholesterol: 3 mg

Chocolate—Peanut Butter Pie

One lovely spring day when their crabapple tree was in full bloom and the lilacs were just coming out, I took one of these pies over to Vera and Aulden Wilson's and we all sat at the kitchen table, along with their guest, Mrs. Emma Strong, and enjoyed it without even thinking that we were deprived because we all, except for Mrs. Strong, have diabetes.

9-inch Graham Cracker Piecrust (page 154)
2 cups fat-free milk
¼ cup chunky peanut butter

1-ounce package reduced-calorie, sugar-free instant chocolate pudding mix
2 cups light whipped topping

Prepare crust and bake. Set aside.

Place milk and peanut butter in mixer bowl and mix at medium speed until well blended. Add pudding mix and mix at medium speed to blend well. When the pudding begins to thicken, pour into the prepared piecrust and refrigerate until firm. Cut into 8 or 10 equal slices and serve 1 slice per serving, garnishing each piece with about 2 tablespoons whipped topping.

Yield: 8 servings
Food exchanges per serving: 1 starch and 1½ fat; or 1 carbohydrate choice
Sugar per serving: 1 teaspoon or 4 grams
Low-cholesterol diets: Use reduced-fat peanut butter and fat-free whipped topping.
Low-sodium diets: Use salt-free margarine when preparing the crust.
Nutritive values per serving:

Calories: 166
CHO: 17 g
PRO: 5 g

FAT: 8 g
Na: 352 mg
Cholesterol: 2 mg

Yield: 10 servings
Food exchanges per serving: 1 starch and 1 fat; or 1 carbohydrate choice
Sugar per serving: .8 teaspoon or 3 grams
Low-cholesterol diets: Use reduced-fat peanut butter and fat-free whipped topping.
Low-sodium diets: Use salt-free margarine when preparing the crust.
Nutritive values per serving:

Calories: 133
CHO: 14 g
PRO: 4 g

FAT: 6 g
Na: 281 mg
Cholesterol: 2 mg

Easy Pineapple Pie

This creamy pie has a light, fruity taste, especially satisfying by itself or after a grilled summer meal.

9-inch Graham Cracker Piecrust (page 154) or 9-inch Shortening Piecrust (page 157)

20-ounce can crushed pineapple in juice or water pack

3.4-ounce package instant lemon pudding and pie filling mix

1 cup very cold fat-free milk

1 cup light whipped topping

1 teaspoon grated lemon peel

1½ tablespoons lemon juice

1 teaspoon lemon extract

Mint leaves and/or lemon twists

Prepare crust and bake. Set aside.

Drain pineapple well. Combine pudding mix and milk in medium bowl. Beat 2 to 3 minutes until very thick. Fold in whipped topping, pineapple, lemon peel, lemon juice, and lemon extract. Pour into crust. Cover and refrigerate 4 hours or overnight. Garnish with mint leaves and/or lemon twists. Cut into 8 or 10 equal pieces.

Yield: 8 servings
Food exchanges per serving: 1½ starch, 1 fruit, and 2 fat; or 2 carbohydrate choices
Sugar per serving: 4.3 teaspoons or 18 grams
Low-cholesterol diets: Recipe is suitable as written.
Low-sodium diets: Omit salt in crust.
Nutritive values per serving:

Calories: 230
CHO: 35 g
PRO: 4 g
FAT: 9 g

Na: 330 mg (graham crust);
936 mg (shortening crust)
Cholesterol: 0

Yield: 10 servings
Food exchanges: 1½ starch and 2 fat; or 2 carbohydrate choices
Sugar per serving: 3.4 teaspoons or 14 grams
Low-cholesterol diets: Recipe is suitable as written.
Low-sodium diets: Omit salt in crust.
Nutritive values per serving:

Calories: 184
CHO: 28 g
PRO: 3 g
FAT: 7 g

Na: 264 mg (graham crust);
749 mg (shortening crust)
Cholesterol: 0

Layered Double-Chocolate Pie

Chocolate fans will savor this easy-to-make, creamy pie that you can prepare in less than 10 minutes.

9-inch Shortening Piecrust (page 157) or 9-inch Graham Cracker Piecrust (page 154)
1-ounce package reduced-calorie, sugar-free instant chocolate pudding mix
1⅓ cups plus 2 tablespoons fat-free milk

½ teaspoon vanilla extract
2 cups light whipped topping
1-ounce package reduced-calorie, sugar-free instant white chocolate pudding mix
1.55-ounce Hershey's milk chocolate candy bar

Prepare crust and bake. Set aside.

In a bowl, mix chocolate pudding mix with ⅔ cup plus 1 tablespoon milk and ¼ teaspoon vanilla until smooth. Stir in half of the whipped topping until well mixed. Pour the pudding mixture into the piecrust and spread evenly.

In another bowl, mix the white chocolate pudding mix with remaining milk and vanilla until smooth. Stir in remaining whipped topping until well blended. Pour the white chocolate mixture over the chocolate pudding mixture and spread evenly. Top pie with chocolate shavings from ¼ of the candy bar. Chill 2 to 4 hours. Cut into 8 or 10 equal slices.

Yield: 8 servings
Food exchanges per serving: 2 starch and 1½ fat; or 2 carbohydrate choices
Sugar per serving: 4.6 teaspoons or 19 grams
Low-cholesterol diets: Recipe is suitable as written.
Low-sodium diets: Omit salt in piecrust. Use your own discretion for inclusion in your diet
Nutritive values per serving:

Calories: 229
CHO: 31 g
PRO: 4 g

FAT: 10.6 g
Na: 41.5 mg
Cholesterol: 1 mg

Yield: 10 servings

Food exchanges per serving: 2 starch and 1 fat; or 1 carbohydrate choice

Sugar per serving: 3.6 teaspoons or 15 grams

Low-cholesterol diets: Recipe is suitable as written.

Low-sodium diets: Omit salt in piecrust. Use your own discretion for inclusion in your diet.

Nutritive values per serving:

Calories: 183   FAT: 8.5 g
CHO: 25 g   Na: 33.2 mg
PRO: 3 g   Cholesterol: 0.5 mg

Lemon Chiffon Pie

This recipe makes a big, impressive pie. If you don't want that much filling, you can remove a cup or two and use it for a separate dessert. (The filling, without the crust, is a free food.) You may also substitute other flavors for the lemon, such as strawberry or orange.

9-inch Graham Cracker Piecrust (page 154)
0.46-ounce package dry lemonade mix sweetened with NutraSweet
0.3-ounce package sugar-free lemon-flavored gelatin

1 cup boiling water
2 tablespoons instant nonfat dry milk
6 (1-gram) packets Equal or Sweet One sugar substitute

Prepare crust and bake. Set aside.

Place lemonade mix and gelatin in a mixer bowl and mix lightly with a spoon. Add boiling water and stir to dissolve. Let cool to room temperature and then refrigerate until syrupy.

Add dry milk and sugar substitute, and beat at high speed for about 5 minutes, or until mixture is creamy and holds a peak. Pour mixture into piecrust and refrigerate until firm. Cut into 8 equal slices.

Yield: 8 servings
Food exchanges per serving: ⅔ starch and 1 fat; or 1 carbohydrate choice
Sugar per serving: 1 teaspoon or 4 grams
Low-cholesterol diets: Recipe is suitable as written.
Low-sodium diets: Use salt-free margarine in crust.
Nutritive values per serving:

Calories: 91
CHO: 9 g
PRO: 3 g

FAT: 5 g
Na: 130 mg
Cholesterol: 0

Sour Cream—Raisin Pie

I had never tasted this pie until we moved to Wadena but you see it frequently at church dinners and potlucks and on restaurant menus here, and I really like it.

9-inch Margarine Piecrust
   (page 156)
2 cups water
2/3 cup raisins
3 large eggs (2 of them
   separated)
3 tablespoons cornstarch

Dry sugar substitute equal to
   1/2 cup sugar
1/8 teaspoon salt
1/2 cup sour cream
2 teaspoons vanilla extract
1/4 teaspoon cream of tartar
1/4 cup sugar

Prepare crust and bake. Set aside.

Place water and raisins in a pan and simmer, covered, for 3 minutes. Cool to lukewarm.

Mix 1 whole egg and 2 egg yolks (reserve 2 egg whites for meringue) with cornstarch, dry sugar substitute, and salt, and blend well. Add sour cream and mix well. Drain liquid from raisins and beat the liquid into sour cream mixture. Cook and stir over medium heat until mixture thickens; then add raisins and vanilla and stir lightly. Cool to room temperature and pour into piecrust.

Beat the 2 reserved egg whites and cream of tartar together at high speed until soft peaks form. Add sugar and continue to beat at high speed to form meringue. Spread meringue evenly over top of pie, making sure that meringue touches crust on all sides. Bake at 350°F for 15 to 20 minutes, or until meringue is lightly browned. Cool on a wire rack to room temperature. Cut into 8 equal slices.

Yield: 8 servings

Food exchanges per serving: 2 starch and 2 fat; or 2 carbohydrate choices

Sugar per serving: 1.5 teaspoons or 6 grams

Low-cholesterol diets: Omit whole egg and egg yolks in filling. Use 1/2 cup liquid egg substitute.

Low-sodium diets: In crust, omit salt and use salt-free margarine.

Nutritive values per serving:

Calories: 238	FAT: 11 g
CHO: 31 g	Na: 200 mg
PRO: 5 g	Cholesterol: 102 mg

Lemon Cream Pie

This lemon cream was my mother's special pie, which she made frequently. It can be made without the lemon rind, but it is much better with grated rind and fresh lemon juice.

9-inch Graham Cracker
 Piecrust (page 154)
1/4 cup cornstarch
2 tablespoons sugar
1/4 teaspoon salt
1/4 cup water at room
 temperature
1/4 cup lemon juice

3/4 cup eggs (about 3 large)
2 cups hot water
Grated rind from 1 lemon
Dry sugar substitute equal
 to 3/4 cup sugar
Diabetic or light
 whipped topping
 (optional)

Prepare crust and bake. Set aside.

Place cornstarch and sugar in mixer bowl and mix at medium speed to blend well. Add salt and room temperature water and mix at medium speed until smooth. Add lemon juice and eggs and mix at medium speed until smooth. Mix in hot water at low speed. Pour mixture into a small pan and cook, stirring, over medium heat until thickened and smooth. Remove from heat and add rind and dry sugar substitute.

Cool about 5 minutes and then spread evenly in crust. Refrigerate until ready to serve and then divide into 8 or 10 equal slices. Garnish with whipped topping if desired.

Yield: 8 servings
Food exchanges per serving: 1 starch and 1 fat; or 1 carbohydrate choice
Sugar per serving: .7 teaspoon or 3 grams
Low-cholesterol diets: Omit eggs. Use 3/4 cup liquid egg substitute. Use fat-free whipped topping as desired.
Low-sodium diets: Omit salt. Use salt-free margarine when preparing the crust. Omit salt in the crust.
Nutritive values per serving:

Calories: 143
CHO: 15 g
PRO: 4 g

FAT: 8 g
Na: 196 mg
Cholesterol: 81 mg

Yield: 10 servings

Food exchanges per serving: 1 starch and 1 fat; or 1 carbohydrate
  choice

Sugar per serving: .6 teaspoon or 2.4 grams

Low-cholesterol diets: Omit eggs. Use ¾ cup liquid egg substitute.
  Use fat-free whipped topping as desired.

Low-sodium diets: Omit salt. Use salt-free margarine when preparing
  the crust. Omit salt in the crust.

Nutritive values per serving:

Calories: 114	FAT: 6 g
CHO: 12 g	Na: 157 mg
PRO: 3 g	Cholesterol: 65 mg

Chocolate Cream Puffs

It is essential that you follow this recipe exactly. The eggs must be at room temperature, and you must use starch flour because it has enough gluten to compensate for the use of cocoa instead of part of the flour. It's a very special dessert, which freezes beautifully and can be thawed in the refrigerator for a special treat.

1 cup water
½ cup (1 stick) margarine
2 tablespoons unsweetened cocoa powder

⅞ cup (14 tablespoons) starch flour
¼ teaspoon cinnamon
3 large eggs at room temperature

Filling

1 cup fat-free milk
1.3-ounce package sugar-free instant chocolate pudding mix

About 1-ounce package sugar-free whipped topping mix or 2 cups light whipped topping

Place water and margarine in a small saucepan; heat over low heat until water is simmering and margarine is melted. Stir cocoa, flour, and cinnamon together to blend. (A good way to measure flour is to put cocoa in a 1-cup measure and fill the rest of the way with flour.) Add flour mixture to hot liquid, and cook, stirring, over medium heat until dough forms a ball around the spoon and pulls away from the sides of the pan. Place ball of dough in a mixer bowl and let stand at room temperature for 5 minutes. Add eggs to dough one at a time, beating well after each addition. Drop dough by 3 tablespoonfuls (level no. 20 dipper) onto a cookie sheet that has been sprayed with cooking spray or lined with aluminum foil.

Bake at 400°F for 30 minutes, or until puffs are firm. Remove from the oven and cut a little slit in the side of each puff with a sharp knife. Return puffs to the oven, turn off the heat, and leave them in the oven for 30 minutes. Then remove puffs from the oven, place on a wire rack, and cool, in a draft-free area, to room temperature.

For filling: Combine milk and pudding mix, blend well, and set aside. Prepare topping according to package directions or use whipped topping. Stir pudding into topping and blend well.

Cut the top off each puff and pull out the soft lining with fingers or a fork. Fill each with a tenth of the filling, about 3 tablespoons. Put the tops back on the puffs and refrigerate until served.

Notes: Various flavorings, such as rum or mint, may be added to the filling for variety.

The filled puffs freeze well for up to 1 month. To serve, remove them from the freezer and place uncovered in the refrigerator an hour or so before use.

Puffs may be sprinkled lightly with powdered sugar, or served with a tablespoon of the same kind of whipped topping used in the filling, without any effect on the food exchange values.

Chocolate Cream Puffs without Filling

Yield: 10 servings (10 cream puffs)
Food exchanges per serving: ⅔ starch and 2 fat; or 1 carbohydrate
    choice
Sugar per serving: None
Low-cholesterol diets: Use fat-free whipped topping. Use your
    discretion for inclusion in your diet.
Low-sodium diets: Use salt-free margarine.
Nutritive values per serving:

Calories: 147	FAT: 10 g
CHO: 10 g	Na: 141 mg
PRO: 3 g	Cholesterol: 76 mg

Chocolate Cream Puffs with Filling

Yield: 10 servings (10 cream puffs)
Food exchanges per serving: 1 starch and 2 fat; or 1 carbohydrate
    choice
Sugar per serving: None
Low-cholesterol diets: Use fat-free whipped topping. Use your
    discretion for inclusion in your diet.
Low-sodium diets: Use salt-free margarine.
Nutritive values per serving:

Calories: 177	FAT: 11 g
CHO: 14 g	Na: 289 mg
PRO: 4 g	Cholesterol: 77 mg

Fran's Cream Puffs

Frances Nielsen, of Oak Lawn, Illinois, has been making these cream puffs for as long as I've known her. She uses this pastry dough, which she, with her European background, calls *pâté à choux*, for appetizers as well as desserts; it's especially delightful when she shapes the dough like little swans. Here, as often in Fran's kitchen, the puffs are filled with pudding and dusted with powdered sugar.

1 cup water	1 cup all-purpose flour
1/4 cup (1/2 stick) margarine	3 large eggs

Filling

About 1-ounce package sugar-free whipped topping mix or 2 cups light whipped topping	1/8 teaspoon salt
	1 cup fat-free milk
1.3-ounce package sugar-free instant vanilla pudding mix	1 teaspoon rum, vanilla, or other flavoring
	2 tablespoons powdered sugar

Place water and margarine in a heavy saucepan; bring to a boil over low heat. Add flour all at once, and cook, stirring with a wooden spoon, over low heat until dough pulls away from the sides of the pan. Place dough in a mixer bowl and let stand at room temperature for 5 minutes. Add eggs to dough one at a time, beating at medium speed after each addition, until glossy; do not overbeat. Drop dough by 3 tablespoonfuls (level no. 20 dipper) onto a cookie sheet that has been sprayed with cooking spray, greased with margarine, or lined with aluminum foil.

Bake at 400°F for 25 minutes; then, without opening the oven door, reduce heat to 350°F and bake for 30 minutes. Remove puffs from the oven and with a sharp knife puncture each one, about where you intend to cut to remove the top; then return to the oven for another 5 minutes. You can test a puff by removing it and letting it sit in a draft-free spot for 2 minutes. If it doesn't fall, puffs are done and can be removed to a wire rack to cool to room temperature. Be careful to let them cool in a place protected from drafts; if they cool too rapidly, they may fall. When puffs are cool, cut off and reserve the tops, and carefully remove any soft dough inside with a spoon.

For filling: Prepare whipped topping according to package directions or use whipped topping and refrigerate until needed. Prepare pudding according to package directions, but use only 1 cup milk, and add your desired flavoring. Refrigerate pudding until firm and then combine with whipped topping. Fill each puff with a tenth of the pudding mixture, about ⅓ cup. Replace tops and dust puffs with powdered sugar. Refrigerate until served.

Note: Unfilled cream puffs should be frozen if you don't plan to use them within 24 hours. They can be defrosted at 250°F in the oven or on low in the microwave oven.

Yield: 10 servings (10 cream puffs with filling)
Food exchanges per serving: 1 starch and 1 fat; or 1 carbohydrate choice
Sugar per serving: 0.3 teaspoon or 1 gram
Low-cholesterol diets: Use fat-free whipped topping. Use your discretion for inclusion in your diet.
Low-sodium diets: Omit salt. Use salt-free margarine.
Nutritive values per serving:

Calories: 191 FAT: 7 g
CHO: 15 g Na: 280 mg
PRO: 4 g Cholesterol: 97 mg

CHAPTER 9

Puddings

THERE ARE SEVERAL very good reduced-calorie, sugar-free commercial puddings on the market. They can be used alone or combined with sugar-free fruit gelatin and/or fruit. There is a place, however, for puddings made from scratch when you can make them. This is especially true at harvest time, when there is an abundance of fresh fruit in your orchard or at the nearest fruit stand or market.

As with all other desserts, the best-quality ingredients are needed for a successful pudding. You should always follow a recipe exactly the first time you prepare it. After that you can vary it, as long as you remember to take into account the nutritive values of the added ingredients when calculating the grams of carbohydrate or exchanges for the final product. For instance, if you add a small banana, which is 15 grams of carbohydrate or 1 fruit exchange, to a vanilla pudding that yields four servings, you must calculate an extra 4 grams of carbohydrate or ¼ fruit exchange for each serving. If you add ¼ cup fresh or frozen blueberries or 1 cup fresh or frozen raspberries to the pudding, calculate an extra 4 grams of carbohydrate or ¼ fruit exchange for each of the four servings.

Puddings made with fruit will add fiber as well as vitamins and minerals to your diet. Custard, bread pudding, and rice pudding are also ideal and often complement a meal without adding excessive carbohydrates or food exchanges.

Baked Custard

This was one of my husband's favorite desserts. I think he could have eaten it two or three times a week and it was good for him, so I made it frequently, using the low-cholesterol version, of course.

2 cups water	¼ teaspoon salt
3 large eggs	Dry sugar substitute equal to
¾ cup instant nonfat dry milk	¼ cup sugar
1½ teaspoons vanilla extract	Nutmeg (optional)

Heat 2 cups water to 110° to 115°F. Place eggs, dry milk, vanilla, salt, and dry sugar substitute in a bowl and mix well. Stir hot water into egg mixture. Blend well, and pour a fourth of mixture into each of four custard cups. Sprinkle custard lightly with nutmeg if desired, and place the cups in an 8- or 9-inch cake pan. Pour boiling water around the cups to a depth of 1½ inches.

Bake at 325°F for about 1 hour, or until a knife comes out clean from the center of custard. Cool at room temperature. Serve warm or chilled.

Yield: 4 servings
Food exchanges per serving: ⅔ milk and 1 fat; or ½ carbohydrate choice
Sugar per serving: None
Low-cholesterol diets: Omit eggs. Use ¾ cup liquid egg substitute.
Low-sodium diets: Omit salt.
Nutritive values per serving:

Calories: 101	FAT: 3 g
CHO: 8 g	Na: 255 mg
PRO: 9 g	Cholesterol: 161 mg

Baked Rice Pudding

Rice pudding is a favorite at our dinner table. This recipe is an ideal way to turn leftover rice into an old-fashioned gourmet delight.

4 cups fat-free milk
½ cup uncooked long-grain rice
¼ cup raisins
2 tablespoons butter or
  margarine
3 large eggs, beaten

⅓ cup sugar
1 teaspoon vanilla extract
½ teaspoon salt
¼ teaspoon nutmeg
¼ teaspoon cinnamon
Light cream or milk

In a heavy, medium saucepan bring 2 cups of the milk, the uncooked rice, and the raisins to a boil. Reduce heat, cover, and cook over very low heat about 15 minutes, or until rice is tender. Remove from heat; stir in butter or margarine until melted.

In a bowl stir together the eggs, the remaining 2 cups milk, and the sugar, vanilla, and salt. Gradually stir rice mixture into egg mixture. Pour into a 10 × 6-inch baking dish.

Bake at 325°F for 25 minutes. Stir well; sprinkle with nutmeg and cinnamon. Bake for an additional 15 to 20 minutes, or until a knife inserted near the center comes out clean. Serve warm or chilled with light cream or milk as desired.

Yield: 8 (½-cup) servings
Food exchanges per serving: 2 starch; or 2 carbohydrate choices
Sugar per serving: 4 teaspoons or 17 grams
Low-cholesterol diets: Use margarine. Omit eggs. Use ¾ cup liquid
  egg substitute.
Low-sodium diets: Omit salt. Use low-salt butter or margarine.
Nutritive values per serving:

Calories: 185
CHO: 27 g
PRO: 8 g

FAT: 5 g
Na: 190 mg
Cholesterol: 89 mg

Bread Pudding

The whole trick in this bread pudding is to use dry bread or toast. You can also use 5 bread exchanges of some other kind of bread such as the Raisin Bread on page 230. My husband liked it made with day-old Italian or French bread.

5 slices commercial white or whole-wheat bread	3 large eggs
2 tablespoons sugar	Dry sugar substitute equal to ¾ cup sugar
¼ teaspoon cinnamon	2 teaspoons vanilla extract
2¾ cups warm water (110° to 115°F)	¼ teaspoon salt
¾ cup instant nonfat dry milk	¼ cup raisins

Toast bread, cool, and cut into cubes. Set aside.

Combine sugar and cinnamon. Set aside.

Place water and dry milk in a bowl; stir to dissolve milk. Add eggs, dry sugar substitute, vanilla, and salt, and beat until well blended. Place half of bread cubes in the bottom of a 9-inch square cake pan that has been sprayed with cooking spray or greased with margarine. Sprinkle raisins evenly over bread cubes; top with remaining bread cubes. Pour milk mixture over bread cubes, and push them down into milk mixture. Sprinkle cinnamon sugar evenly over bread cubes.

Bake at 325°F for 50 to 60 minutes, or until a knife comes out clean from center of pudding. Cool on a wire rack in a draft-free area. Cut pudding three by three.

Note: This pudding is good warm or refrigerated. I generally serve it with part of my milk exchange.

Yield: 9 servings
Food exchanges per serving: 1 starch and ½ fat; or 1 carbohydrate choice
Sugar per serving: .7 teaspoon or 3 grams
Low-cholesterol diets: Omit eggs. Use ¾ cup liquid egg substitute. Egg whites do not yield a satisfactory pudding.
Low-sodium diets: Omit salt.
Nutritive values per serving:

Calories: 107	FAT: 2 g
CHO: 16 g	Na: 191 mg
PRO: 5 g	Cholesterol: 71 mg

Chocolate Pudding

¼ cup sugar
2 tablespoons cornstarch
⅛ teaspoon salt
2 squares (2 ounces)
  unsweetened chocolate,
  chopped
2 cups fat-free milk

2 beaten egg yolks, 1 beaten egg,
  or ½ cup egg substitute
1 tablespoon butter or
  margarine
1½ teaspoons vanilla extract
Dry sugar substitute equal to ¼
  to ½ cup sugar

In a heavy, medium saucepan combine sugar, cornstarch, salt, and chocolate. Stir in milk. Cook, stirring, over medium heat until thickened and bubbly. Cook, stirring, 2 minutes more. Remove from heat. Gradually stir about 1 cup of the hot mixture into egg yolks. Return mixture to saucepan. Cook, stirring, 2 minutes. Remove from heat. Stir in butter, vanilla, and sugar substitute to taste. Pour into a bowl. Cover surface with clear plastic wrap. Chill without stirring. To serve, spoon pudding into individual dishes.

Yield: 4 (½-cup) servings
Food exchanges per serving: 1 starch, 1 milk, and 2 fat; or 2
  carbohydrate choices
Sugar per serving: 4.3 teaspoons or 18 grams
Low-cholesterol diets: Omit eggs. Use ½ cup liquid egg substitute.
  Omit unsweetened chocolate and substitute ¼ cup low-fat,
  unsweetened cocoa powder.
Low-sodium diets: Omit salt. Use salt-free margarine.
Nutritive values per serving:

Calories: 260	FAT: 13 g
CHO: 29 g	Na: 180 mg
PRO: 8.5 g	Cholesterol: 108 mg

Creamy Chocolate Pudding

Garnish with a dollop of light whipped cream.

1/4 cup sugar
Dry sugar substitute equal to 5
tablespoons plus 1½
teaspoons sugar
3 tablespoons all-purpose flour
1 tablespoon cornstarch
1/8 teaspoon salt

1/4 cup unsweetened cocoa
powder
1/3 cup instant nonfat dry
milk
2 cups fat-free milk
2 tablespoons margarine
1 teaspoon vanilla extract

In a saucepan, mix sugar, dry sugar substitute equal to 5 tablespoons sugar, flour, cornstarch, salt, cocoa, and dry milk. Add fat-free milk and mix well. Cook, stirring constantly, over medium heat until mixture thickens, about 5 minutes. Remove from heat and add margarine, vanilla, and dry sugar substitute equal to 1½ teaspoons sugar. Stir until smooth.

Pour into serving dishes. Cover with plastic wrap and cool completely.

Yield: 5 (½-cup) servings
Food exchanges per serving: 2 starch; or 2 carbohydrate choices
Sugar per serving: 4 teaspoons or 17 grams
Low-cholesterol diets: Recipe is suitable as written.
Low-sodium diets: Omit salt. Use salt-free margarine.
Nutritive values per serving:

Calories: 149
CHO: 26 g
PRO: 6 g

FAT: 3 g
Na: 176 mg
Cholesterol: 3 mg

Creamy Orange Pudding

1/4 cup cornstarch
1/4 cup sugar
1/4 teaspoon salt
1/2 cup orange juice
2 large eggs
2 1/4 cups boiling water
1 tablespoon margarine

1 teaspoon orange flavoring
Grated rind from 1 orange
Dry sugar substitute equal to
   1/4 cup sugar
About 1-ounce package sugar-
   free whipped topping mix or
   1 cup light whipped topping

Place cornstarch, sugar, salt, orange juice, and eggs in a mixer bowl and mix at medium speed until smooth, scraping down the bowl once during the mixing. Pour water over orange juice mixture and beat until smooth. Pour mixture into a saucepan, add margarine, and cook, stirring, over medium heat for 2 minutes, or until mixture is thickened and smooth and starchy taste is gone. Remove pudding from heat and add flavoring, rind, and sugar substitute. Chill pudding, and pour 1/2 cup into each of six serving dishes. Prepare whipped topping according to package directions or use whipped topping and garnish pudding when it is served.

Note: A piece of plastic wrap over the pudding will prevent a skin from forming on it while it is chilling.

Yield: 6 (1/2-cup) servings
Food exchanges per serving: 1 starch and 1 fat; or 1 carbohydrate
   choice
Sugar per serving: 2 teaspoons or 8 grams
Low-cholesterol diets: Omit eggs. Use 1/2 cup egg whites or liquid egg
   substitute.
Low-sodium diets: Omit salt. Use salt-free margarine.
Nutritive values per serving:

Calories: 126	(without whipped topping, 104)
CHO: 15 g	FAT: 4 g
PRO: 2 g	Na: 134 mg
	Cholesterol: 91 mg

Fruit Gelatin

Most of us know how to prepare fruit gelatin, but I wanted to include directions for counting the carbohydrate grams or exchanges when we add fruit to sugar-free gelatin. In order to calculate the carbohydrate grams or exchanges in a serving of fruit gelatin, add up the number of carbohydrate grams or fruit exchanges you have used and divide by the number of servings. For instance, if you add 1 cup drained, sugar-free canned peach slices to 2 cups of gelatin (prepared from a .3-ounce package), you have added 30 grams of carbohydrate or 2 fruit exchanges to your gelatin. Therefore you divide the 30 carbohydrate grams or 2 fruit exchanges by 4, the number of servings, and you have 7.5 grams of carbohydrate or ½ fruit exchange in each ½-cup serving of fruit gelatin. (Check your fruit exchange list to find the food exchange values for the various fruits.) Nutritive values for peach gelatin are as follows:

Yield: 4 (½-cup) servings
Food exchanges per serving: ½ fruit; or ½ carbohydrate choice
Sugar per serving: None
Low-cholesterol diets: Recipe is suitable as written.
Low-sodium diets: Recipe is suitable as written.
Nutritive values per serving:

Calories: 32	FAT: 1 g
CHO: 6 g	Na: 70 mg
PRO: 2 g	Cholesterol: 0

Applesauce and cranberry sauce have a high water content and should be considered liquids when used in gelatin. Dissolve a .3-ounce packet of sugar-free fruit-flavored gelatin in 1 cup boiling water, add 1 cup applesauce or cranberry sauce to the dissolved gelatin mixture, and chill until firm. This will yield 2 cups gelatin, or 4 ½-cup servings, with ½ fruit exchange or 7.5 grams of carbohydrate for each serving made with applesauce. Unsweetened cranberry sauce is free up to ½ cup, so the cranberry gelatin will be a free food.

Lemon Cream Pudding

The freshly squeezed lemon juice gives this pudding a tart, zesty, and refreshing flavor. It's so delicious you'll never want to use instant varieties again. Garnish with whipped topping and a lemon twist.

¼ cup sugar
¼ cup cornstarch
⅛ teaspoon salt
¼ cup lemon juice (preferably fresh squeezed)
2 large egg yolks, slightly beaten

1½ cups hot water
Dry sugar substitute equal to ¼ cup sugar
1 teaspoon lemon extract
Grated rind from 1 lemon

In a small saucepan mix sugar and cornstarch together until well blended. Add salt, lemon juice, and egg yolks and mix well using a wire whisk. Add hot water and mix until smooth. Cook, stirring, over medium heat until thickened and smooth, about 5 minutes.

Remove from heat and add sugar substitute, lemon extract, and lemon rind. Pour into individual dishes. Cover with plastic wrap to prevent a skin from forming. Cool before serving.

Yield: 4 (½-cup) servings
Food exchanges per serving: 1 starch and ½ fruit; or 1½ carbohydrate choice
Sugar per serving: 3.1 teaspoons or 13 grams
Low-cholesterol diets: Omit eggs. Use ½ cup liquid egg substitute.
Low-sodium diets: Omit salt.
Nutritive values per serving:

Calories: 110	FAT: 1.5 g
CHO: 23 g	Na: 15 mg
PRO: 2 g	Cholesterol: 55 mg

Ozark Pudding

Kay Knochel, from Phoenix, Arizona gave me this recipe when we were sharing an apartment not long after we both graduated from college. She suggested I include it in this book because we both like it so much; we think other people will too. Serve warm or at room temperature with Orange Sauce (page 199).

¼ cup all-purpose flour	¼ teaspoon salt
1½ teaspoons baking powder	2 large eggs
⅓ cup sugar	1 teaspoon vanilla extract
Dry sugar substitute equal to	¼ cup chopped walnuts
½ cup sugar	1 cup chopped fresh tart apples

Place flour, baking powder, sugar, dry sugar substitute, and salt in a mixer bowl and mix at low speed for 30 seconds to blend well. Stir eggs and vanilla together with a fork and add to flour mixture. Mix at medium speed only until flour is moistened. Add walnuts and apples and mix lightly. Spread pudding evenly in an 8-inch square baking pan that has been sprayed with cooking spray or greased with margarine.

Bake at 350°F for 30 to 35 minutes, or until pudding is lightly browned and pulls away from the sides of the pan. Cool on a wire rack. Cut pudding two by three.

Yield: 6 servings
Food exchanges per serving: 1 starch, ⅔ fruit, and 1 fat; or 2 carbohydrate choices
Sugar per serving: 2.5 teaspoons or 10 grams
Low-cholesterol diets: Omit eggs. Use ½ cup liquid egg substitute.
Low-sodium diets: Omit salt. Use low-sodium baking powder.
Nutritive values per serving:

Calories: 127	FAT: 5 g
CHO: 26 g	Na: 195 mg
PRO: 5 g	Cholesterol: 127 mg

Pineapple Pudding

Serve warm or chilled with Lemon Sauce (page 199).

¼ cup packed brown sugar
Dry brown sugar substitute
   equal to ¼ cup brown
   sugar
¼ teaspoon cinnamon
¼ cup chopped walnuts
1 cup all-purpose flour
¼ cup sugar

Dry sugar substitute equal to
   ½ cup sugar
1 teaspoon baking soda
¼ teaspoon salt
15¼-ounce can crushed
   pineapple in its own juice
¼ teaspoon almond extract
1 large egg

Combine brown sugar, dry brown sugar substitute, cinnamon, and walnuts, and mix to blend. Set aside.

Place flour, sugar, dry sugar substitute, baking soda, and salt in a mixer bowl and mix at low speed to blend well. Stir together pineapple, flavoring, and egg, and add to flour mixture. Mix at medium speed until blended. Spread batter evenly in a 9-inch square cake pan that has been sprayed with cooking spray or greased with margarine. Sprinkle reserved brown sugar mixture evenly over batter.

Bake at 350°F for about 40 minutes, or until pudding is browned and a cake tester comes out clean from the center. Cool on a wire rack. Cut pudding three by three.

Yield: 9 servings
Food exchanges per serving: 1 starch, 1 fruit, and ½ fat; or 2
   carbohydrate choices
Sugar per serving: 2.7 teaspoons or 11 grams
Low-cholesterol diets: Omit egg. Use ¼ cup egg whites or liquid egg
   substitute.
Low-sodium diets: Omit salt.
Nutritive values per serving:

        Calories: 156   FAT: 3 g
        CHO: 30 g   Na: 183 mg
        PRO: 3 g   Cholesterol: 28 mg

Pumpkin Pecan Pudding

I generally use a part of my milk exchange on this pudding. It adds a creamy taste to the pudding, although the pudding is also good alone.

16-ounce can solid pack pumpkin

12-ounce can evaporated fat-free milk

1/3 cup packed brown sugar

2 large eggs

1 to 2 teaspoons pumpkin pie spice

Dry sugar substitute equal to 1/4 cup sugar

1/2 teaspoon salt

1 teaspoon vanilla extract

1/2 cup chopped pecans

Place pumpkin, milk (add enough water to it to equal 1½ cups, if necessary), brown sugar, eggs, pumpkin pie spice, dry sugar substitute, salt, and vanilla in a mixer bowl and mix at medium speed until smooth and creamy. Pour into an 8-inch square baking pan that has been sprayed with cooking spray or greased with margarine. Sprinkle pecans evenly over top of pudding.

Bake at 325°F (300°F if you are using a glass baking dish) for about 1 hour, or until a knife comes out clean from the center of the pudding. Cool to room temperature. Cut three by four.

Yield: 12 servings

Food exchanges per serving: 1 starch and 1 fat; or 1 carbohydrate choice

Sugar per serving: 1.3 teaspoons or 5 grams

Low-cholesterol diets: Omit eggs. Use 1/2 cup egg whites or liquid egg substitute.

Low-sodium diets: Omit salt.

Nutritive values per serving:

Calories: 105   FAT: 4 g

CHO: 14 g   Na: 142 mg

PRO: 4 g   Cholesterol: 47 mg

Raspberry Trifle

I always think of my friends Bud and Frances Gunsallus when I make this dessert. Bud discovered trifle on a trip to England, and we have enjoyed it ever since, using different-flavored gelatins and different fruits for variety.

0.3-ounce package sugar-free
   raspberry-flavored gelatin
1 cup boiling water
1 cup cold water
1 cup unsweetened fresh or
   frozen red raspberries

1-ounce package sugar-free
   instant vanilla pudding mix
1¾ cups fat-free milk
1 medium banana
¼ cup sweetened, flaked
   coconut

Dissolve gelatin in boiling water; add cold water and raspberries. Pour into a 9-inch square cake pan. Refrigerate until firm.

Combine pudding mix and milk, and beat together to blend. Slice banana and stir it gently into pudding. Pour pudding evenly over firm gelatin and refrigerate until firm. Sprinkle coconut evenly over pudding and refrigerate pudding until served. Cut three by three.

Note: I prepare this pudding in a glass dish if I'm going to take it to a potluck dinner or buffet; it looks especially good that way.

Yield: 9 servings
Food exchanges per serving: ⅔ starch; or 1 carbohydrate choice
Sugar per serving: None
Low-cholesterol diets: Recipe is suitable as written. Low-sodium diets:
   Recipe is suitable as written.
Nutritive values per serving:

Calories: 56
CHO: 11 g
PRO: 2 g

FAT: 0
Na: 195 mg
Cholesterol: 0

Rice Pudding

This is an easy version of rice pudding, but you'd never know when you are eating it.

2 cups fat-free milk
1-ounce package sugar-free
  instant vanilla pudding mix
½ teaspoon vanilla extract

Dry sugar substitute equal to
  ⅓ cup sugar
1 cup cooked rice,
  drained

Stir milk and pudding mix together until smooth. Add vanilla and dry sugar substitute, and mix lightly. Add rice and mix lightly. Refrigerate until served.

Note: This pudding may be garnished with a sprinkle of cinnamon, a couple of chocolate chips, or a fresh strawberry, a couple of cherries or raspberries, or other bits of fruit.

Yield: 5 (½-cup) servings
Food exchanges per serving: 1 starch; or 1 carbohydrate choice
Sugar per serving: None
Low-cholesterol diets: Recipe is suitable as written. Instant dry milk
  does not generally yield a good pudding.
Low-sodium diets: Cook rice without salt.
Nutritive values per serving:

Calories: 74
CHO: 16 g
PRO: 4 g

FAT: 0
Na: 267 mg
Cholesterol: 0

Tapioca Pudding

This recipe is based on one from Chef Dave Hutchins, of Cedar Rapids. I asked him once why his tapioca pudding was so good—I generally don't like tapioca—and he told me it was because he added more eggs and sugar and jazzed it up, which I try to do.

2¼ cups water
½ cup instant nonfat dry milk
2 large eggs
2 tablespoons sugar
3 tablespoons quick-cooking tapioca

Dry sugar substitute equal to ¼ cup sugar
1½ teaspoons vanilla extract
1 or 2 drops yellow food coloring

Combine water, dry milk, eggs, and sugar in a saucepan and beat with a whip or beater until smooth. Add tapioca, stir lightly, and let stand for 5 minutes. Then cook, stirring, over medium heat until mixture comes to a full boil. Remove from heat and add dry sugar substitute, vanilla, and food coloring. Stir lightly; let cool at least 20 minutes or to room temperature and then refrigerate or serve.

Note: Garnish this pudding with a sprinkling of cinnamon, a cube of sugar-free fruit gelatin, or a bit of fresh fruit, such as a strawberry or a few fresh cherries or blueberries.

Yield: 6 (½-cup) servings
Food exchanges per serving: 1 milk; or 1 carbohydrate choice
Sugar per serving: 1 teaspoon or 4 grams
Low-cholesterol diets: Omit eggs. Use ½ cup liquid egg substitute.
Low-sodium diets: Recipe is suitable as written.
Nutritive values per serving:

Calories: 77
CHO: 11 g
PRO: 6 g

FAT: 2 g
Na: 64 mg
Cholesterol: 87 mg

Vanilla Pudding

Traditional homemade vanilla pudding is a hands-down favorite any-time.

¼ cup sugar
2 tablespoons cornstarch
⅛ teaspoon salt
2 cups fat-free milk
2 beaten egg yolks, 1 beaten egg, or ½ cup liquid egg substitute

1 tablespoon butter or margarine
1½ teaspoons vanilla extract
Dry sugar substitute equal to 8 teaspoons sugar

In a heavy, medium saucepan combine sugar, cornstarch, and salt. Stir in milk. Cook, stirring, over medium heat until thickened and bubbly. Cook, stirring, 2 minutes more. Remove from heat. Gradually stir about 1 cup of the hot mixture into egg yolks. Return mixture to saucepan. Cook, stirring, 2 minutes. Remove from heat. Stir in butter, vanilla, and sugar substitute to taste. Pour into a bowl. Cover surface with clear plastic wrap. Chill without stirring. To serve, spoon pudding into individual dishes.

Yield: 4 (½-cup) servings
Food exchanges per serving: 1 milk and 1 starch; or 1½ carbohydrate choices
Sugar per serving: 4.3 teaspoons or 18 grams
Low-cholesterol diets: Instead of eggs, use the ½ cup liquid egg substitute.
Low-sodium diets: Omit salt. Use salt-free margarine.
Nutritive values per serving:

Calories: 179   FAT: 5 g
CHO: 24 g   Na: 180 mg
PRO: 8 g   Cholesterol: 108 mg

Whipped Gelatin

Since this whipped gelatin is free, I use it in many ways: as a topping for other gelatins and for cooled cakes, as a layer in parfaits, as a dessert garnished with fruit (you must count the fruit in your daily exchanges), as a filling for a graham cracker crust in a low-calorie pie, or just as a dessert.

0.3-ounce package sugar-free
  fruit-flavored gelatin
1 cup boiling water
¼ cup cold water

2 tablespoons instant nonfat dry
  milk
Dry sugar substitute equal to
  ¼ cup sugar

Stir gelatin and boiling water together until gelatin is dissolved. Add cold water, and place mixture in a mixer bowl. Chill until gelatin is syrupy. Add dry milk and dry sugar substitute to gelatin and beat at high speed, using a whip, for about 5 minutes, or until gelatin is creamy and holds a peak. Chill until firm and use as desired.

Note: It's better to prepare the gelatin within 2 or 3 hours of the time it is to be served, because it eventually loses its volume. Any flavor of fruit gelatin may be used, and appropriate fruit may be added or may garnish the dessert. You must take into account the additional exchange and nutritive values of any fruit used.

Yield: 8 (1-cup) servings
Food exchanges per serving: Free up to 4 cups
Sugar per serving: None
Low-cholesterol diets: Recipe is suitable as written.
Low-sodium diets: Recipe is suitable as written.
Nutritive values per serving:

Calories: 8
CHO: .5 g
PRO: 1 g

FAT: 0
Na: 35 mg
Cholesterol: 0

Blueberry Sauce

This sauce is good on ice milk, ice cream, frozen yogurt, plain cake, and pudding. I also like to add it to my cereal and milk in the morning.

3 cups unsweetened
   fresh or frozen
   blueberries
3 cups water
2 tablespoons cornstarch

1 tablespoon lemon juice
1 tablespoon margarine
Dry sugar substitute equal to
   ½ cup sugar
¼ teaspoon salt

Combine blueberries and water in a saucepan, cover, and simmer for 10 minutes. Drain well, reserving the juice. Place drained blueberries and cornstarch, along with ½ cup of the blueberry juice, in a food processor and blend until smooth. Combine blended mixture with remaining juice in a saucepan, and cook, stirring, until thickened. Remove from heat and add lemon juice, margarine, dry sugar substitute, and salt. Stir until margarine is melted. Serve warm or chilled. Makes 3 cups.

Yield: 12 (¼-cup) servings
Food exchanges per serving: ½ fruit; or ½ carbohydrate choice
Sugar per serving: None
Low-cholesterol diets: Recipe is suitable as written.
Low-sodium diets: Omit salt. Use salt-free margarine.
Nutritive values per serving:

Calories: 36
CHO: 7 g
PRO: 1 g

FAT: 1 g
Na: 56 mg
Cholesterol: 0

Chocolate Sauce

You can vary this sauce by substituting different flavorings such as peppermint, rum, or cherry for the vanilla.

2 cups water
2 tablespoons instant nonfat dry milk
2 tablespoons cornstarch
¼ cup unsweetened cocoa powder

¼ teaspoon salt
1 tablespoon margarine
2 teaspoons vanilla extract
Dry sugar substitute equal to ½ cup sugar

Put 1 cup of the water in a small saucepan, cover, and bring to a boil. Put remaining 1 cup water in a small bowl with dry milk, cornstarch, cocoa, and salt, and beat with a hand beater or blend in a food processor until smooth. Add boiling water and mix well. Pour the mixture into the saucepan, add margarine, and cook, stirring constantly, over medium heat until mixture simmers. Cook and simmer over low heat for 1 to 2 minutes, or until the starchy taste is gone. Remove from heat. Add vanilla and dry sugar substitute, and mix lightly. Cool to room temperature. Makes 2 cups.

Yield: 8 (¼-cup) servings
Food exchanges per serving: 1 vegetable; or no carbohydrate choices
Sugar per serving: None
Low-cholesterol diets: Recipe is suitable as written.
Low-sodium diets: Omit salt. Use salt-free margarine.
Nutritive values per serving:

Calories: 31
CHO: 4 g
PRO: 1 g

FAT: 2 g
Na: 106 mg
Cholesterol: 0

Dark Chocolate Sauce

This very versatile sauce is one I like to make when my friends Butch and Jan Franks and their son, John, come over for the evening. They love ice cream and I enjoy giving it to them with this topping and all its variations.

1 cup water
2 tablespoons instant nonfat dry milk
1 tablespoon cornstarch
¼ cup sugar
¼ cup unsweetened cocoa powder
⅛ teaspoon salt
⅓ cup light corn syrup
2 tablespoons margarine
Dry sugar substitute equal to ½ cup sugar
1 teaspoon vanilla extract

Bring water to a boil in a saucepan. Stir dry milk, cornstarch, sugar, cocoa, and salt together to blend and add to the boiling water. Cook over medium heat, stirring with a wire whip, until smooth. Add corn syrup and margarine and simmer over low heat, stirring frequently, for 2 minutes or until thickened. Add sugar substitute. Remove from heat and add vanilla. Cool to room temperature and refrigerate until needed or up to 3 days. Return to room temperature before serving. Makes 2 cups.

Yield: 16 (2-tablespoon) servings
Food exchanges per serving: 1 starch; or 1 carbohydrate choice
Sugar per serving: 1.7 teaspoons or 7 grams
Low-cholesterol diets: Recipe is suitable as written.
Low-sodium diets: Omit salt and use salt-free margarine. Use reduced-sodium peanut butter in the Chocolate Peanut Butter Sauce.
Nutritive values per serving:

Calories: 50   FAT: 1.5 g
CHO: 10 g   Na: 45 mg
PRO: 0   Cholesterol: 0

Variations: Light Chocolate Sauce: Reduce cocoa to 3 tablespoons and increase dry milk to ⅓ cup.

Semisweet Chocolate Sauce: Increase cocoa to ⅓ cup and omit cornstarch.

Chocolate Peanut Butter Sauce: Beat ½ cup peanut butter into the sauce just before it is served.

Chocolate Nut Sauce: Add 1 cup chopped nuts to the sauce just before it is served.

Chocolate Cherry Sauce: Add 1 cup chopped maraschino cherries to the sauce just before it is served.

Chocolate Peppermint Sauce: Add 1 teaspoon peppermint flavoring along with the vanilla.

Custard Sauce

This sauce complements fresh fruit, fruit gelatin, and gingerbread, among other things. It is good warm, lukewarm, or chilled, depending upon how and when you plan to use it. It is especially good on baked apples, using chilled sauce and warm apples, or warm sauce and chilled apples, and it is very good on ginger and other spice cakes.

2 cups water
⅓ cup instant nonfat dry milk
¼ cup sugar
2 tablespoons cornstarch
⅛ teaspoon salt
2 teaspoons margarine

¼ cup liquid egg substitute
3 drops yellow food coloring
Dry sugar substitute
    equivalent to 2 teaspoons
    sugar
1½ teaspoons vanilla extract

Combine water, dry milk, sugar, cornstarch, and salt in a small saucepan and stir until smooth. Add the margarine and cook over medium heat, stirring constantly, until thickened and smooth. Remove from the heat. Beat about ½ cup sauce into the egg substitute. Return mixture to the saucepan and bring to a simmer, stirring constantly. Remove from the heat, add food coloring, sugar substitute, and vanilla and mix lightly.

Serve warm, lukewarm, or chilled. Refrigerate sauce if it will not be used within 30 minutes. Makes 2¼ cups.

Variation: Rum Custard Sauce: Decrease vanilla to 1 teaspoon and add 1 teaspoon rum flavoring.

Yield: 9 (¼-cup) servings
Food exchanges per serving: 1 starch; or 1 carbohydrate choice
Sugar per serving: 1.7 teaspoons or 7 grams
Low-cholesterol diets: Recipe is suitable as written.
Low-sodium diets: Omit salt. Use low-sodium margarine.
Nutritive values per serving:

Calories: 50
CHO: 9 g
PRO: 2 g

FAT: 1 g
Na: 70 mg
Cholesterol: 0

Orange Sauce

I like to prepare food from scratch because I can control the amount of carbohydrate in the food, but I also like to take advantage of some of the prepared foods, such as sugar substitutes, sugar-free drinks, gelatins, and puddings, because I know they contain ingredients I couldn't buy.

2¼ cups water
2 tablespoons cornstarch

1 to 2 teaspoons dry sugar-free orange-flavored drink mix

Stir water and cornstarch together in a small saucepan until cornstarch is dissolved. Cook, stirring frequently, over medium heat until clear. Continue to stir over low heat for another minute, or until the starchy taste is gone. Remove from heat. Add drink mix, using as much as needed to get the desired taste. Serve warm or cold over cake or pudding. Makes 2 cups.

Variations: Lemon Sauce: Substitute dry sugar-free lemonade mix for orange drink mix. There is no effect on the nutritive values or exchanges.

Cinnamon Sauce: Omit orange drink mix and substitute 1 teaspoon ground cinnamon, 1 teaspoon vanilla, and dry sugar substitute equal to ½ cup sugar. There is no effect on the nutritive values or exchanges.

Yield: 8 (¼-cup) servings
Food exchanges per serving: ¼ cup is free; ½ cup (2 servings) is 1 vegetable exchange or no carbohydrate choice.
Sugar per serving: None
Low-cholesterol diets: Recipe is suitable as written.
Low-sodium diets: Recipe is suitable as written.
Nutritive values per serving:

Calories: 10	FAT: 0
CHO: 2 g	Na: 0
PRO: 0	Cholesterol: 0

CHAPTER 10

$\mathcal{S}$weet $\mathcal{B}$reads
and $\mathcal{M}$uffins

A VARIETY OF breads can add interest and variety to your diet. When using bakery breads, check the label carefully. These delicious products often come in serving sizes two to three times the average portion and are frequently high in fats and sugars.

Like many people, I enjoy muffins or coffee cake for breakfast; I also enjoy special breads for toast and sandwiches. The time spent making them is worth it, as I hope you will discover. If you don't have time to prepare yeast breads, you might try muffins or the hot breads; they aren't difficult, and they add a lot to your menus.

Here are some special things to remember when you are making bread:

1. You must use exactly the kind of flour specified in the recipe. I like to use bread flour in bread recipes because it is higher in protein (gluten) and makes a better loaf of bread. However, bread flour needs more liquid than all-purpose flour, so you can't substitute one for the other without changing the amount of liquid and the final yield and exchange and carbohydrate values will also be affected.

I also enjoy making breads with different kinds of flour. I'm a firm believer in a high-fiber diet, so I often use whole-wheat, cracked-wheat, and/or bran in breads. I keep these flours in airtight containers in the freezer until just before I need them, in order to keep them fresh, and I always bring them back to room temperature before using them but they stay better in the freezer unless you intend to use them soon. I keep them in plastic or glass gallon jars but you can keep them in any airtight freezer container.

2. The temperature of the water or liquid you use to dissolve the yeast in is very important. Because yeast is a living plant, too much heat can kill its action, while not enough heat can slow it down. Active dry yeast is best dissolved in liquid at 105° to 115°F. I recommend using an instant-read thermometer to check the temperature of the liquid. If you do not have a thermometer, drop a little liquid on the inside of your wrist. It should feel comfortably warm, but not hot. Using a thermometer, however, is the best method for ensuring a proper liquid temperature for dissolving the yeast. Of all your "must-have" kitchen tools, a thermometer is one of the most important and is useful in almost all types of cooking.

3. Instant nonfat dry milk is used frequently in these recipes. It is good for yeast breads because it doesn't have to be scalded. It is easy to store and generally less expensive than regular milk; in addition, it softens the texture of breads, helps them brown in the oven, and will give them a softer crust.

4. The dough hook on your mixer can be a great help when making breads. If you don't have a dough hook, the bread can be mixed by hand, but you must be careful to knead it sufficiently to develop the gluten in the flour. My mother used to tell about the woman she knew who kneaded her bread for an hour. I thought that was silly but it does take a good ten minutes of kneading to develop the gluten in the bread flour.

5. Bread machines take much of the work out of making bread. To adapt a recipe for use in your home bread machine, place all the ingredients into the container as recommended in your owner's manual. Typically, liquid ingredients are placed in the bottom of the container with dry ingredients on top. The yeast is usually placed in the center of the flour just before beginning the mixing process. Follow the manufacturer's instructions for baking.

6. All of your equipment should be very clean when you are preparing breads, especially yeast breads, since bacteria can affect the flavor and taste of bread. I like to use nonstick bread pans, and spray them with cooking spray, because the bread comes out of the pan more easily. It is important to use the pan size specified in the recipe if you want a standard product.

7. Sugar in the dough helps the texture of breads, as well as the flavor. It also helps breads brown well. Sugar substitutes can yield a loaf that is less browned or more dense and less soft than a loaf made with sugar. All of the recipes used here will give good results with the use of less sugar or sugar substitutes. It is especially important, however, that you follow the directions closely. In some recipes, fruits can also be used to enhance the bread's flavor.

Blueberry Coffee Cake

I use blueberries frequently in muffins, pancakes, and cakes—and in this coffee cake, a family favorite.

2 tablespoons brown sugar
Dry brown sugar substitute equal to ¼ cup brown sugar
½ teaspoon cinnamon
¼ cup (½ stick) margarine at room temperature
¼ cup sugar
Dry sugar substitute equal to ¼ cup sugar

2 large eggs
1½ cups all-purpose flour
¼ cup instant nonfat dry milk
1 tablespoon baking powder
½ teaspoon salt
¾ cup water
1 cup unsweetened fresh or frozen blueberries

Stir brown sugar, dry brown sugar substitute, and cinnamon together well. Set aside.

Cream margarine, sugar, and dry sugar substitute together at medium speed until light and fluffy. Add eggs and mix at medium speed to blend, scraping down the bowl before and after addition. Stir flour, dry milk, baking powder, and salt together to blend well. Add to creamed mixture along with water. Mix at medium speed only until flour is moistened. Add blueberries. Spread batter evenly in a 9-inch square cake pan that has been sprayed with cooking spray or greased with margarine. Sprinkle brown sugar-cinnamon mixture on top.

Bake at 375°F for about 40 minutes, or until cake is lightly browned and a cake tester comes out clean from the center. Remove to a wire rack. Cut three by four. Serve warm or at room temperature.

Yield: 12 servings
Food exchanges per serving: 1 starch, ⅓ fruit, and 1 fat; or 1 carbohydrate choice
Sugar per serving: 1.5 teaspoons or 6 grams
Low-cholesterol diets: Omit eggs. Use ½ cup egg whites or liquid egg substitute.
Low-sodium diets: Omit salt. Use salt-free margarine and low-sodium baking powder.
Nutritive values per serving:

Calories: 136	FAT: 4 g
CHO: 20 g	Na: 238 mg
PRO: 3 g	Cholesterol: 38 mg

Czech Coffee Cake

This rather porous coffee cake makes excellent toast. I generally use it for a breakfast treat, although you might enjoy it as an afternoon snack with coffee.

1 envelope (2¼ teaspoons) Rapid Rise active dry yeast
1 teaspoon sugar
¾ cup water at 110° to 115°F
2¼ cups bread flour
¼ cup instant nonfat dry milk
Dry brown sugar substitute equal to ½ cup brown sugar

2 tablespoons margarine at room temperature
2 large eggs
½ teaspoon salt
½ teaspoon mace
1 teaspoon lemon flavoring
Grated rind of 1 large lemon or 1 tablespoon finely chopped dried lemon peel

Place yeast and sugar in a mixer bowl and stir lightly. Add water and let stand for 5 to 10 minutes, or until foamy. Add 1 cup of the flour and mix at medium speed (use a dough hook) for 4 minutes. Add dry milk, dry brown sugar substitute, margarine, eggs, salt, mace, lemon flavoring and rind, and remaining flour. Mix at medium speed for 4 minutes. Spread dough evenly (it will be sticky) in a 9 × 5-inch loaf pan that has been sprayed with cooking spray or greased with margarine. Cover the pan with wax paper and a clean cloth, and let dough rise until almost to the top of the pan.

Bake at 350°F for about 45 minutes, or until cake is browned and firm. Remove to a wire rack. Cut into 16 (½-inch) slices. Serve warm.

Yield: 16 servings
Food exchanges per serving: 1 starch; or 1 carbohydrate choice
Sugar per serving: Negligible
Low-cholesterol diets: Omit eggs. Use ½ cup egg whites or liquid egg substitute.
Low-sodium diets: Omit salt. Use salt-free margarine.
Nutritive values per serving:

Calories: 90
CHO: 14 g
PRO: 3 g

FAT: 1 g
Na: 98 mg
Cholesterol: 30 mg

Dessert Crêpes

The cherry filling is very good with these crêpes, but you may use other fillings as long as you take into account the altered nutritive values and exchanges.

	Vanilla	Chocolate
Cake flour	1 cup	1 cup
Cocoa	—	1/4 cup
Sugar	1/4 cup	2 tablespoons
Baking soda	1/8 teaspoon	1/8 teaspoon
Fat-free milk	1 1/8 cups	1 1/4 cups
Large eggs	2	2
Vegetable oil	2 tablespoons	3 tablespoons
Vanilla extract	1 teaspoon	1 teaspoon
Melted margarine	As necessary	As necessary
Cherry Filling (page 206)	1 3/4 cups	1 3/4 cups
Powdered sugar	2 tablespoons	2 tablespoons

Stir dry ingredients together to blend well. Mix milk, eggs, oil, and vanilla together with a fork to blend well. Add mixture to dry ingredients and beat until smooth. Cover and refrigerate from 4 hours to overnight.

It is best to use a special crêpe pan for preparing crêpes. I prefer the 6- or 8-inch pans with a nonstick lining; I use them only for frying crêpes, and I season them beforehand. Chef Walter Marion, with whom I worked at Swift & Company in Chicago, always insisted crêpe pans should be wiped out with a paper towel and never washed in soapy water. If you do wash them in soapy water, you should season them again before using them.

Preheat the pan until a drop of water sizzles in it. Brush the pan lightly with a paper towel dipped in melted margarine, and pour about 2 1/2 tablespoons batter into the pan. Rotate the pan as soon as you add batter so it will cover the bottom of the pan. Let crêpe cook for 1 minute, and then turn it over and cook it about 30 seconds on the other side. I generally cook crêpes over medium heat on my stove and you will soon learn which heat setting is best for crêpes on your stove. Turn each crêpe out onto a clean paper towel or plate. Crêpes can be stacked on an ovenproof plate or baking dish and kept warm in the oven at about 200°F.

Fill each warm crêpe with 2 tablespoons Cherry Filling. Roll each up and sprinkle lightly with powdered sugar.

Note: Crêpes can be prepared ahead of time and frozen with wax paper or aluminum foil between them. They will keep, tightly wrapped, in the freezer for up to 6 weeks. They should be thawed in their wrappings in the refrigerator or at room temperature and can be reheated at 350°F for 8 to 10 minutes. They may then be filled as desired.

Yield: 14 servings (14 crêpes)
Low-cholesterol diets: Omit eggs. Use ½ cup liquid egg substitute.
Low-sodium diets: Recipe is suitable as written.

Nutritive values for Vanilla Crêpes
Sugar per serving: .9 teaspoon or 4 grams

	Without filling	With filling
Calories:	79	101
CHO:	11 g	16 g
PRO:	3 g	3 g
FAT:	3 g	3 g
Na:	30 mg	32 mg
Cholesterol:	37 mg	37 mg
Food exchanges per serving:	⅔ starch, 1 fat; or 1 carbohydrate choice	1 starch, 1 fat; or 1 carbohydrate choice

Nutritive values for Chocolate Crêpes
Sugar per serving: .6 teaspoon or 2.5 grams

	Without filling	With filling
Calories:	91	113
CHO:	12 g	17 g
PRO:	3 g	3 g
FAT:	4 g	4 g
Na:	42 mg	44 mg
Cholesterol:	37 mg	37 mg
Food exchanges per serving:	⅔ starch, 1 fat; or 1 carbohydrate choice	1 starch, 1 fat; or 1 carbohydrate choice

Cherry Filling for Crêpes

This can be used as a filling for other things such as Chocolate Cream Puffs (page 174), or as a topping for ice cream, ice milk, frozen yogurt, or plain cake or pudding.

16-ounce can water-packed red tart cherries
Dry sugar substitute equal to ¼ cup sugar
Water as necessary

1 tablespoon cornstarch
¼ cup sugar
⅛ teaspoon almond flavoring
2 drops red food coloring (optional)

Drain cherries well, reserving liquid. Sprinkle dry sugar substitute over cherries, mix lightly, and set aside. Add water, if necessary, to reserved liquid to yield a total of 1 cup. Add cornstarch and sugar to liquid, stir until smooth, and then cook, stirring, over medium heat for 3 to 4 minutes, or until thickened and the starchy taste is gone. Remove from heat. Add flavoring and food coloring (if using), and stir lightly. Add cherries and stir lightly. Use immediately or refrigerate until needed.

Note: ⅓ cup plus 2 teaspoons filling is equal to 1 fruit exchange.

Yield: 16 (2-tablespoon) servings
Food exchanges per serving: ⅓ fruit; or ⅓ carbohydrate choice
Sugar per serving: .8 teaspoon or 3 grams
Low-cholesterol diets: Recipe is suitable as written.
Low-sodium diets: Recipe is suitable as written.
Nutritive values per serving:

Calories: 22
CHO: 5 g
PRO: Negligible

FAT: 0
Na: 2 mg
Cholesterol: 0

Kringla

This recipe came from my cousin Therese Ballantine, of Ames, Iowa. Although she isn't Scandinavian, she grew up in North Dakota and collected many of the wonderful Scandinavian recipes in use there. These are a cross between bread and cookies, and they are generally served with coffee or tea. They are very good warm, but I also like them cold.

½ cup (1 stick) margarine at room temperature
¾ cup sugar
Dry sugar substitute equal to ¼ cup sugar (optional)
1 large egg

1 teaspoon vanilla extract
3¼ cups all-purpose flour
1 teaspoon baking soda
1 teaspoon baking powder
1 cup sour cream

Cream together margarine, sugar, and dry sugar substitute (if using) at medium speed until light and fluffy. Add egg and vanilla, and mix at medium speed until creamy. Stir flour, baking soda, and baking powder together to blend; add, along with sour cream, to creamy mixture. Mix at medium speed until blended. Turn dough out onto a floured work surface and knead a few times until smooth. Shape dough into a ball, place in a bowl, cover, and refrigerate from 3 hours to overnight.

After refrigerating, divide dough into 2 equal portions. Roll each out on a floured surface to form a 12 × 4-inch oblong. Cut each portion of the dough into 16 equal pieces about 4 × ¾ inches. Roll each piece in your hands or on the work surface to form a rope 8 inches long. Shape ropes of dough into wreaths or figure eights. Place dough on cookie sheets that have been sprayed with cooking spray or greased lightly with margarine.

Place them in an oven that has been preheated to 400°F, turn the heat down to 350°F, and bake for about 15 minutes, or until browned on the bottom and very lightly browned on top. Remove to a wire rack. Serve hot or warm.

Note: These may be brushed with milk or an egg-white-and-water mixture before they are baked, for a crisper crust. Doing so does not affect the exchange values.

Yield: 32 servings
Food exchanges per serving: 1 starch and 1 fat; or 1 carbohydrate choice
Sugar per serving: 1.1 teaspoons or 4.5 grams
Low-cholesterol diets: Omit egg. Use ¼ cup egg whites or liquid egg substitute.
Low-sodium diets: Recipe is suitable as written.
Nutritive values per serving:

Calories: 107	FAT: 5g
CHO: 15 g	Na: 75 mg
PRO: 2 g	Cholesterol: 12 mg

Raisin Bran Coffee Cake

This recipe is based on one from my cousin Virginia Ballantine, of Clarion, Iowa. I've always enjoyed it, so I took out some of the sugar and adapted it for my diet.

2 tablespoons sugar
¼ teaspoon cinnamon
1 cup all-purpose flour
2 tablespoons instant nonfat dry
   milk
1 tablespoon baking powder
Dry sugar substitute equal to
   ¼ cup sugar (optional)

¼ teaspoon salt
1½ cups All-Bran, Bran Buds,
   Fiber One, or 100% Bran
⅓ cup raisins
1 cup water
2 large eggs
⅓ cup vegetable oil
1 teaspoon vanilla extract

Stir sugar and cinnamon together to blend well. Set aside.

Place flour, dry milk, baking powder, dry sugar substitute (if using), salt, cereal, and raisins in a mixer bowl; mix at low speed to blend well. Stir water, eggs, oil, and vanilla together to blend well; add to flour mixture. Mix at medium speed only until flour is moistened. Pour batter into a 9-inch square cake pan that has been sprayed with cooking spray or greased with margarine. Sprinkle cinnamon sugar evenly over batter.

Bake at 350°F for 30 to 35 minutes, or until cake pulls away from the sides of the pan and springs back when touched in the center. Cut four by four. Serve warm, if possible.

Yield: 16 servings
Food exchanges per serving: 1 starch and 1 fat; or 1 carbohydrate choice
Sugar per serving: .4 teaspoon or 2 grams
Low-cholesterol diets: Omit eggs. Use ½ cup egg whites or liquid egg substitute.
Low-sodium diets: Omit salt. Use low-sodium baking powder.
Nutritive values per serving:

Calories: 109
CHO: 14 g
PRO: 3 g

FAT: 6 g
Na: 259 mg
Cholesterol: 34 mg

Sour Cream Coffee Cake

This recipe is adapted from the classic sour cream coffee cake we have all been making for years.

¼ cup (½ stick) margarine at room temperature
¼ cup packed brown sugar
Dry brown sugar substitute equal to ½ cup brown sugar
2 large eggs
1 cup reduced-fat sour cream

1 teaspoon vanilla extract
2 cups all-purpose flour
½ teaspoon baking soda
½ teaspoon baking powder
½ teaspoon salt
1 teaspoon cinnamon
¼ cup water at room temperature

Cream margarine, brown sugar, and dry brown sugar substitute at medium speed until light and fluffy. Add eggs, sour cream, and vanilla, and mix at medium speed until creamy, scraping down the bowl before and after adding them. Stir flour, baking soda, baking powder, salt, and cinnamon together to blend, and add, along with water, to creamy mixture. Mix at medium speed until creamy. Spread batter evenly in a 9-inch square cake pan that has been sprayed with cooking spray or greased with margarine.

Bake at 375°F for 25 to 30 minutes, or until cake is lightly browned and a cake tester comes out clean from the center. Cut four by four. Serve hot or at room temperature.

Yield: 16 servings
Food exchanges per serving: 1 starch and 1 fat; or 1 carbohydrate choice
Sugar per serving: .8 teaspoon or 3 grams
Low-cholesterol diets: Omit eggs. Use ½ cup liquid egg substitute. May also want to use fat-free sour cream.
Low-sodium diets: Omit salt. Use salt-free margarine and low-sodium baking powder.
Nutritive values per serving:

Calories: 138
CHO: 16 g
PRO: 3 g

FAT: 4 g
Na: 154 mg
Cholesterol: 20 mg

Strawberry-Rhubarb Coffee Cake

I make this cake in the spring, when rhubarb is in season; it isn't as good made with frozen rhubarb.

2 cups fresh rhubarb cut into
½-inch pieces
3-ounce package strawberry-flavored fruit gelatin (not sugar-free)
Dry sugar substitute equal to ½ cup sugar
¼ cup (½ stick) margarine at room temperature
⅓ cup sugar

1 large egg
1 teaspoon vanilla extract
1 cup all-purpose flour
1 cup All-Bran, Bran Buds, Fiber One, or 100% Bran
1 tablespoon baking powder
⅛ teaspoon salt
2 tablespoons instant nonfat dry milk
1 cup water

Place rhubarb in a bowl. Stir gelatin and half the dry sugar substitute (equal to ¼ cup sugar) together and mix with rhubarb. Set aside.

Cream margarine, sugar, and remaining dry sugar substitute together at medium speed until light and fluffy. Add egg and vanilla, and mix at medium speed for 30 seconds, scraping down the bowl before and after addition. Stir flour, cereal, baking powder, salt, and dry milk together to blend well; add, along with water, to creamy mixture. Mix at medium speed only until flour is moistened. Spread batter evenly in a 9-inch square cake pan that has been sprayed with cooking spray or greased with margarine. Spread reserved rhubarb mixture, including any liquid or powder left in the bowl, evenly over batter.

Bake at 375°F for about 40 minutes, or until cake starts to pull away from the sides of the pan and a cake tester comes out clean from the center. Remove the pan to a wire rack. Cut four by four. Serve warm or at room temperature.

Yield: 16 servings
Food exchanges per serving: 1 starch, ⅔ fruit, and 1 fat; or 2 carbohydrate choices
Sugar per serving: 2 teaspoons or 8 grams
Low-cholesterol diets: Omit egg. Use ¼ cup egg whites or liquid egg substitute.
Low-sodium diets: Omit salt. Use salt-free margarine and low-sodium baking powder.
Nutritive values per serving:

Calories: 140
CHO: 24 g
PRO: 3 g

FAT: 5 g
Na: 202 mg
Cholesterol: 21 mg

Applesauce Oat Bran Muffins

These luscious muffins contain two good sources of fiber: applesauce and oat bran.

1 cup oat bran cereal
1 cup all-purpose flour
1 teaspoon baking soda
2 tablespoons dry buttermilk
1/2 cup packed brown sugar
1/4 teaspoon salt
1 teaspoon cinnamon or apple pie spice
1/2 cup raisins
1 cup unsweetened applesauce
1/4 cup vegetable oil
1 large egg

Place oat bran, flour, baking soda, dry buttermilk, brown sugar, salt, spice, and raisins in a mixer bowl; mix at low speed for 30 seconds to blend well. Stir applesauce, oil, and egg together to blend, and add to flour mixture. Mix at medium speed until creamy. Fill the cups of a 12-muffin pan that has been sprayed with cooking spray, lined with paper liners, or greased with margarine, halfway with batter (level no. 20 dipper).

Bake at 400°F for 18 to 20 minutes, or until muffins are browned and the centers spring back when touched. Serve warm.

Yield: 12 muffins
Food exchanges per muffin: 1 starch, 1 fruit, and 1 fat; or 2 carbohydrate choices
Sugar per muffin: 2 teaspoons or 8 grams
Low-cholesterol diets: Omit egg. Use 1/4 cup egg whites or liquid egg substitute.
Low-sodium diets: Omit salt.
Nutritive values per muffin:

Calories: 177
CHO: 29 g
PRO: 3 g
FAT: 6 g
Na: 131 mg
Cholesterol: 24 mg

Basic Oat Bran Muffins

As you can see, I'm a firm believer in oat bran. I've seen some really remarkable results in lowering cholesterol counts when oat bran was added to the diet. I include it in my own diet as often as possible, so I have quite a variety of oat bran muffin recipes in my personal file.

¾ cup all-purpose flour
1½ cups oat bran cereal
2 tablespoons sugar
Dry sugar substitute equal to
¼ cup sugar (optional)
1 teaspoon cinnamon

1 teaspoon baking soda
1 cup water at room
temperature
¼ cup vegetable oil
1 tablespoon lemon juice
2 large eggs

Place flour, oat bran, sugar, dry sugar substitute (if using), cinnamon, and baking soda in a mixer bowl and mix at low speed to blend. Stir water, oil, lemon juice, and eggs together with a fork; add to flour mixture. Mix at medium speed until creamy. Fill the cups of a 12-muffin pan that has been sprayed with cooking spray, lined with paper liners, or greased with margarine, halfway with batter (level no. 20 dipper).

Bake at 400°F for 18 to 20 minutes, or until muffins are browned and the centers spring back when touched. Serve warm.

Yield: 12 muffins
Food exchanges per muffin: 1 starch and 1 fat; or 1 carbohydrate choice
Sugar per muffin: .5 teaspoon or 2 grams
Low-cholesterol diets: Omit eggs. Use ½ cup egg whites or liquid egg substitute.
Low-sodium diets: Recipe is suitable as written.
Nutritive values per muffin:

Calories: 128
CHO: 15 g
PRO: 3 g

FAT: 6 g
Na: 81 mg
Cholesterol: 46 mg

Blueberry Oat Bran Muffins

Blueberries are a great favorite of my cousin John Sniffin, who lives in Savage, Minnesota. We are very fond of him, so I try to have his favorite foods available when he comes to visit.

1 cup all-purpose flour
1 cup oat bran cereal
1/3 cup sugar
1/4 cup instant nonfat dry milk
1 teaspoon baking soda
1/4 teaspoon salt

1 cup water
1/3 cup vegetable oil
1 tablespoon lemon juice
1/4 cup egg whites
1 teaspoon vanilla extract
1 cup unsweetened fresh or frozen blueberries

Place flour, cereal, sugar, dry milk, baking soda, and salt in a mixer bowl and mix at low speed for 30 seconds to blend. Stir water, oil, lemon juice, egg whites, and vanilla together with a fork to blend; add to flour mixture. Mix at medium speed until creamy; then add blueberries and mix lightly. Fill the cups of a 12-muffin pan that has been sprayed with cooking spray, lined with paper liners, or greased with margarine, two-thirds full with batter (level no. 16 dipper).

Bake at 400°F for 20 to 22 minutes, or until muffins are lightly browned and the centers spring back when touched. Serve warm.

Yield: 12 muffins
Food exchanges per muffin: 1 starch, 1 fat, and 1/3 fruit; or 1 carbohydrate choice
Sugar per muffin: 1.3 teaspoons or 5 grams
Low-cholesterol diets: Recipe is suitable as written.
Low-sodium diets: Omit salt.
Nutritive values per muffin:

Calories: 153
CHO: 20 g
PRO: 3 g

FAT: 6 g
Na: 130 mg
Cholesterol: 0

Date Bran Muffins

So many of my friends have asked for this recipe that I decided it was worth all of the exchanges and carbohydrate choices. These muffins are like those big dark ones you get at the bakery.

1½ cups all-purpose flour
1½ cups All-Bran, Bran Buds, Fiber One, or 100% Bran
⅓ cup chopped, pitted dates
2 tablespoons instant nonfat dry milk
1 teaspoon baking soda
1 teaspoon baking powder
¼ teaspoon salt
Dry brown sugar substitute equal to ¼ cup brown sugar
1½ cups water
⅓ cup vegetable oil
⅓ cup molasses
1 large egg

Place flour, cereal, dates, dry milk, baking soda, baking powder, salt, and dry brown sugar substitute in a mixer bowl and mix at low speed for 30 seconds to blend well. Stir water, oil, molasses, and egg together with a fork to blend; add to flour mixture. Mix at medium speed until creamy. Fill the cups of a 12-muffin pan that has been sprayed with cooking spray, lined with paper liners, or greased with margarine, two-thirds full with batter (level no. 16 dipper).

Bake at 400°F for 20 to 22 minutes, or until muffins spring back when touched in the center. Serve warm.

Yield: 12 muffins
Food exchanges per muffin: 1 starch, ⅔ fruit, and 1 fat; or 2 carbohydrate choices
Sugar per muffin: Equivalent of 1.3 teaspoons or 5 grams
Low-cholesterol diets: Omit egg. Use ¼ cup egg whites or liquid egg substitute.
Low-sodium diets: Omit salt. Use low-sodium baking powder.
Nutritive values per muffin:

Calories: 170
CHO: 26 g
PRO: 3 g
FAT: 7 g
Na: 239 mg
Cholesterol: 23 mg

Ginger Muffins

If you like molasses cookies made with ginger, you'll love these muffins. I often make them and several other kinds of muffins at the same time, then put a variety in a container in the freezer. That way I don't have to eat the same kind of muffin for days in a row.

1 cup all-purpose flour	Dry brown sugar substitute
1 cup oat bran cereal	equal to ¼ cup brown sugar
¼ teaspoon salt	1 cup water
1 teaspoon baking soda	¼ cup molasses
½ teaspoon ginger	1 large egg
½ teaspoon cinnamon	¼ cup vegetable oil

Place flour, oat bran, salt, baking soda, ginger, cinnamon, and dry brown sugar substitute in a mixer bowl and mix at low speed to blend. Combine water, molasses, egg, and oil, and beat with a fork to blend well. Add to flour mixture and mix at medium speed to blend. Fill the cups of a 12-muffin pan that has been sprayed with cooking spray, lined with paper liners, or greased with margarine, halfway with batter (level no. 20 dipper).

Bake at 400°F for 18 to 20 minutes, or until muffins are firm in the center. Serve warm or freeze for later use.

Yield: 12 muffins
Food exchanges per muffin: 1 starch and 1 fat; or 1 carbohydrate choice
Sugar per muffin: 1 teaspoon or 4 grams
Low-cholesterol diets: Omit egg. Use ¼ cup egg whites or liquid egg substitute.
Low-sodium diets: Omit salt.
Nutritive values per muffin:

Calories: 125	FAT: 6 g
CHO: 16 g	Na: 125 mg
PRO: 3 g	Cholesterol: 23 mg

Mandarin Orange Muffins

¼ cup (½ stick) margarine at room temperature
¼ cup sugar
Dry sugar substitute equal to ¼ cup sugar
1 large egg
1 teaspoon orange flavoring
1 cup all-purpose flour

1¼ cups All-Bran, Bran Buds, Fiber One, or 100% Bran
1 tablespoon baking powder
2 tablespoons instant nonfat dry milk
½ cup water
1 cup well-drained canned mandarin oranges

Cream margarine, sugar, and dry sugar substitute together at medium speed until light and fluffy. Add egg and flavoring, and mix at medium speed for 30 seconds, scraping down the bowl before and after addition. Stir flour, cereal, baking powder, and dry milk together to blend well; add, along with water, to egg mixture. Mix at medium speed only until flour is absorbed. Stir mandarin oranges into batter. Fill the cups of a 12-muffin pan that has been sprayed with cooking spray, lined with paper liners, or greased with margarine, halfway with batter (level no. 20 dipper).

Bake at 400°F for 20 to 22 minutes, or until muffins are lightly browned. Serve hot.

Yield: 12 muffins
Food exchanges per muffin: 1 starch and 1 fat; or 1 carbohydrate choice
Sugar per muffin: 1 teaspoon or 4 grams
Low-cholesterol diets: Omit egg. Use ¼ cup egg whites or liquid egg substitute.
Low-sodium diets: Use salt-free margarine and low-sodium baking powder.
Nutritive values per muffin:

Calories: 117   FAT: 4 g
CHO: 18 g   Na: 203 mg
PRO: 3 g   Cholesterol: 23 mg

Sweet Oat Bran Muffins

I emphasize oat bran when I'm counseling anyone about a carbohydrate-controlled or low-cholesterol diet, because I have found it very helpful to me and others.

1 cup all-purpose flour
1 cup oat bran cereal
2 tablespoons sugar
¼ cup dry buttermilk
Dry brown sugar substitute
  equal to ¼ cup brown sugar

1 teaspoon baking soda
1 cup water
1 large egg
¼ cup vegetable oil
1 teaspoon vanilla
  extract

Place flour, cereal, sugar, dry buttermilk, dry brown sugar substitute, and baking soda in a mixer bowl and mix at low speed to blend well. Combine water, egg, oil, and vanilla, and beat with a fork to blend well. Add liquid to flour mixture and mix at medium speed until creamy. Fill the cups of a 12-muffin pan that has been sprayed with cooking spray, lined with paper liners, or greased with margarine, about halfway with batter (level no. 20 dipper).

Bake at 400°F for about 20 minutes, or until a cake tester comes out clean from the center of a muffin. Serve warm.

Yield: 12 muffins
Food exchanges per muffin: 1 starch and 1 fat; or 1 carbohydrate
  choice
Sugar per muffin: .5 teaspoon or 2 grams
Low-cholesterol diets: Omit egg. Use ¼ cup egg whites or liquid egg
  substitute.
Low-sodium diets: Recipe is suitable as written.
Nutritive values per muffin:

Calories: 129
CHO: 16 g
PRO: 3 g

FAT: 6 g
Na: 88 mg
Cholesterol: 25 mg

Sweet Wheat Bran Muffins

1¼ cups all-purpose flour
1¼ cups All-Bran, Bran Buds,
  Fiber One, or 100% Bran
2 tablespoons sugar
Dry sugar substitute equal to
  ¼ cup sugar (optional)

1 tablespoon baking powder
¼ cup instant nonfat dry milk
1 teaspoon cinnamon
1¼ cups water
1 large egg
¼ cup vegetable oil

Place flour, cereal, sugar, dry sugar substitute (if using), baking powder, dry milk, and cinnamon in a mixer bowl and mix at low speed to blend well. Stir water, egg, and oil together with a fork to blend; add to flour mixture. Mix at medium speed only until flour is moistened. Fill the cups of a 12-muffin pan that has been sprayed with cooking spray, lined with paper liners, or greased with margarine, halfway with batter (level no. 20 dipper).

Bake at 400°F for about 20 minutes, or until muffins are browned and firm. Serve hot.

Yield: 12 muffins
Food exchanges per muffin: 1 starch and 1 fat; or 1 carbohydrate choice
Sugar per muffin: .5 teaspoon or 2 grams
Low-cholesterol diets: Omit egg. Use ¼ cup egg whites or liquid egg substitute.
Low-sodium diets: Use low-sodium baking powder.
Nutritive values per muffin:

Calories: 123
CHO: 17 g
PRO: 3 g

FAT: 7 g
Na: 163 mg
Cholesterol: 23 mg

Zucchini Muffins

Summer zucchini squash makes these muffins a healthy choice for breakfast, snacks, or with a meal. As an added benefit, these muffins freeze well, so you can enjoy the tastes of summer into the fall.

3 cups all-purpose flour	¼ cup unpacked brown sugar
1 teaspoon baking powder	¾ cup vegetable oil
1 teaspoon baking soda	¼ cup unsweetened applesauce
½ teaspoon salt	2 cups grated zucchini
1 teaspoon cinnamon	1 teaspoon vanilla extract
4 large eggs	¼ cup raisins
¾ cup granulated sugar	1 cup chopped nuts (optional)

Combine flour, baking powder, baking soda, salt, and cinnamon in a bowl. Set aside.

Beat eggs and sugars on medium speed for 2 minutes. Slowly add oil, mixing only slightly. Add applesauce and mix well. Add zucchini and vanilla and mix well. Add flour mixture and stir until combined. Stir in raisins and nuts (if using). Do not overmix. Fill 30 cups of muffin pans that have been sprayed with cooking spray, lined with paper liners, or greased with margarine, two-thirds full with batter (level no. 16 dipper).

Bake at 350°F for 25 to 30 minutes. Let stand for 10 minutes before serving.

Yield: 30 muffins

Food exchanges per muffin: 1 starch and 1 fat; or 1 carbohydrate choice

Sugar per serving: 1.9 teaspoons or 8 grams

Low-cholesterol diets: Omit eggs. Use 1 cup egg whites or liquid egg substitute.

Low-sodium diets: Use salt-free margarine and low-sodium baking powder.

Nutritive values per serving:

Calories: 127	FAT: 6 g
CHO: 18 g	Na: 65 mg
PRO: 2 g	Cholesterol: 15 mg

Chocolate Chip Rolls

Children and adults in France and other European countries eat these rolls frequently for snacks and after-school treats. We enjoy them occasionally for breakfast, with coffee and fruit.

2 tablespoons sugar
Dry sugar substitute equal to
   ¼ cup sugar
1¼ cups water at 110° to
   115°F
1 envelope (2¼ teaspoons)
   Rapid Rise active dry
   yeast
2 drops yellow food coloring
   (optional)

3½ cups all-purpose
   flour
1 teaspoon salt
1 egg white
3 tablespoons margarine
   at room temperature
Dry sugar substitute equal
   to ¼ cup sugar (optional)
¾ cup semisweet chocolate
   chips

Combine sugar and ¼ cup dry sugar substitute in a small bowl and stir to blend. Set aside.

Place water in a mixer bowl, add yeast, and let stand for 5 to 10 minutes, or until foamy. Add food coloring (if using) and 2 cups of the flour; mix at medium speed (use a dough hook) for 4 minutes. Add salt, egg white, 1 tablespoon of the margarine, dry sugar substitute (if using), and remaining 1½ cups flour. Continue to mix at medium speed for 2 minutes, or until dough pulls away from the sides of the bowl. Turn dough out onto a floured work surface and knead a few times. Form into a ball and place in a bowl that has been greased with margarine; turn the ball over to grease the top. Cover the bowl with a clean cloth and let dough rise until doubled in volume. Knead dough lightly, form into a ball, and let rest for 10 minutes.

While dough is resting, use a little of the remaining 2 tablespoons of the margarine to grease a 9 × 13-inch cake pan. Sprinkle half of the sugar mixture evenly over the bottom of the pan. Set aside.

Roll dough out onto a lightly floured work surface to form a 14 × 9-inch rectangle. Spread remaining margarine evenly over dough, leaving a clear rim about ½ inch wide all around. Sprinkle remaining sugar mixture evenly over dough, and then chocolate chips evenly over sugar mixture. Shape dough into a 14-inch roll, like a jelly roll. Cut into 14 equal slices 1 inch wide; place these cut side down in the cake pan. Cover the pan with a clean cloth and let dough rise at room temperature until doubled in volume.

Bake at 375°F for about 45 minutes, or until rolls are golden brown. Turn rolls out of the pan onto a wire rack. Serve warm.

Yield: 14 rolls
Food exchanges per roll: 2 starch and 1 fat; or 2 carbohydrate choices
Sugar per serving: .4 teaspoon or 3 grams
Low-cholesterol diets: Recipe is suitable as written.
Low-sodium diets: Omit salt. Use salt-free margarine.
Nutritive values per roll:

Calories: 189	FAT: 5 g
CHO: 30 g	Na: 187 mg
PRO: 4 g	Cholesterol: 0

Banana Bread

Banana bread is a quick and easy way to use leftover bananas. This bread is a nice change of pace from toast for breakfast and sweet enough for an after-dinner dessert. It also freezes well, so I often make an extra loaf to keep on hand for company, gift giving, or a special treat.

1¾ cups all-purpose flour
1¼ teaspoons baking powder
½ teaspoon baking soda
½ cup sugar
¼ cup vegetable shortening or margarine

2 large eggs
2 tablespoons fat-free milk
½ teaspoon vanilla extract
1 cup mashed, ripe bananas

Stir together flour, baking powder, and baking soda. Set aside.

Beat sugar and shortening at medium speed until light and fluffy, scraping sides of bowl often. Add eggs, one at a time, with the milk, beating until smooth after each addition. Add vanilla. Add flour mixture and banana alternately to creamed mixture, beating until smooth after each addition. Turn batter into an 8 × 4-inch loaf pan that has been sprayed with cooking spray.

Bake at 325°F for 50 to 55 minutes, or until a wooden pick inserted near center comes out clean. Cool in pan for 10 minutes. Remove from pan and cool. For easier slicing wrap in plastic wrap and store overnight. Cut into 20 equal slices.

Variation: Chocolate Chip Banana Bread: Chocolate lovers may want to add ¼ cup chocolate chips to the batter before baking. This addition will add 1.3 grams of carbohydrate and 10 calories per slice.

Yield: 20 (1-slice) servings
Food exchanges per serving: 1 starch and ½ fat; or carbohydrate choice
Sugar per serving: 1.75 teaspoons or 7.3 grams
Low-cholesterol diets: Omit eggs. Use ½ cup liquid egg substitute.
Low-sodium diets: Use low-sodium baking powder.
Nutritive values per serving:

Calories: 99
CHO: 17 g
PRO: 2 g

FAT: 3 g
Na: 105 mg
Cholesterol: 21 mg

Orange Pumpkin Bread

1 cup canned solid pack
   pumpkin
2 large eggs
⅓ cup vegetable oil
1 teaspoon orange flavoring
¼ cup sugar
2 tablespoons dry orange-
   flavored breakfast drink mix
   (not sugar-free)

1½ cups all-purpose flour
1 teaspoon baking soda
¼ cup chopped pecans
Dry sugar substitute equal to
   ¼ cup sugar

Place pumpkin, eggs, oil, flavoring, sugar, and drink mix in a mixer bowl; mix at medium speed until creamy. Stir flour, baking soda, pecans, and dry sugar substitute together to blend well, and add to pumpkin mixture. Mix at medium speed until creamy. Spread dough evenly in a 9 × 5-inch loaf pan that has been sprayed with cooking spray or greased with margarine.

Bake at 375°F for about 45 minutes, or until bread pulls away from the sides of the pan and a cake tester comes out clean from the center. Remove pan to a wire rack for 10 minutes, and then turn loaf out onto the rack to cool to room temperature. Cut into 16 equal slices ½ inch wide.

Yield: 16 (1-slice) servings
Food exchanges per serving: 1 starch and 1 fat; or 1 carbohydrate
   choice
Sugar per serving: 1.2 teaspoons or 5 grams
Low-cholesterol diets: Omit eggs. Use ½ cup egg whites or liquid egg
   substitute.
Low-sodium diets: Recipe is suitable as written.
Nutritive values per serving:

Calories: 126	FAT: 7 g
CHO: 15 g	Na: 61 mg
PRO: 2 g	Cholesterol: 34 mg

Orange Cinnamon Bread

This festive Greek bread is generally baked in round loaves. If you want to do it the traditional way, form the bread into two balls, put them in well-greased 8-inch round cake pans, and bake as directed in the recipe.

2 cups hot water
1/3 cup dry orange-flavored breakfast drink mix (not sugar-free)
1/4 cup instant nonfat dry milk
Dry sugar substitute equal to 1/3 cup sugar
1 envelope (2 1/4 teaspoons) Rapid Rise active dry yeast

5 1/4 cups bread flour
2 teaspoons orange flavoring
1 large egg
2 teaspoons salt
1 tablespoon cinnamon
1/3 cup (2/3 stick) margarine at room temperature

Place water, drink mix, dry milk, and dry sugar substitute in a mixer bowl; stir to dissolve drink mix. Cool to 110° to 115°F. Add yeast and let stand for 5 to 10 minutes, or until foamy. Add 2 cups of the flour and mix at medium speed (use a dough hook) for 4 minutes. Add flavoring, egg, salt, cinnamon, margarine, and 3 cups of the flour, and mix for another 4 minutes at medium speed.

Sprinkle remaining 1/4 cup flour on a work surface and turn dough out onto the flour. Knead lightly, using as much flour as necessary to form a smooth, resilient dough. Form dough into a ball and place in a bowl that has been sprayed with cooking spray or greased with margarine. Sprinkle remaining flour from the work surface over dough. Cover the bowl with a clean cloth and let dough rise at room temperature until doubled in volume.

Turn dough out onto a lightly floured work surface and divide into two equal portions. Form each into a ball, place on a lightly floured work surface, cover with a clean cloth, and let rest for 10 minutes. Then shape each ball into a loaf and place each in a 9 × 5-inch loaf pan that has been sprayed with cooking spray or greased with margarine. Cover each pan with a clean cloth and let dough rise until doubled in volume.

Bake at 350°F for 1 hour, or until bread is golden brown. Remove to a wire rack and cool to room temperature. Cut each loaf into 18 equal slices 1/2 inch wide.

Yield: 36 (1-slice) servings
Food exchanges per serving: 1 starch; or 1 carbohydrate choice
Sugar per serving: .4 teaspoon or 2 grams
Low-cholesterol diets: Omit egg. Use ¼ cup egg whites or liquid egg
   substitute.
Low-sodium diets: Omit salt. Use salt-free margarine.
Nutritive values per serving:

Calories: 92	FAT: 1 g
CHO: 16 g	Na: 43 mg
PRO: 2 g	Cholesterol: 4 mg

Pumpkin Bread

This lightly spiced pumpkin bread complements roast pork or turkey. It is especially delicious when also accompanied by cooked cranberries.

½ cup plus 2 tablespoons water at 70° to 80°F
½ cup canned solid pack pumpkin
3 tablespoons butter or margarine at room temperature
¼ cup instant nonfat dry milk powder

3 tablespoons brown sugar
1 teaspoon ground cinnamon
½ teaspoon ground nutmeg
½ teaspoon salt
⅛ teaspoon ground ginger
2¾ cups bread flour
1 envelope (2¼ teaspoons) active dry yeast

In bread machine pan, place all ingredients in order suggested by manufacturer. Select basic bread setting. Choose crust color and select 1½-pound loaf size if available. Bake according to bread machine directions.

Yield: 16 (1-slice) servings
Food exchanges per serving: 1 starch; or 1 carbohydrate choice
Sugar per serving: .7 teaspoon or 3 grams
Low-cholesterol diets: Recipe is suitable as written.
Low-sodium diets: Recipe is suitable as written.
Nutritive values per serving:

Calories: 106
CHO: 19 g
PRO: 3 g

FAT: 2 g
Na: 105 mg
Cholesterol: 0

Chocolate Sweet Bread

This recipe is a favorite of my friend Patti Dillon and her family. Patti was the Fayette County (Iowa) Extension Office home economist. She has been a tremendous help to me with my cookbooks over the past years.

1 tablespoon brown sugar
1 envelope (2¼ teaspoons)
   Rapid Rise active dry yeast
1 cup water at 110° to 115°F
2¼ cups bread flour
2 large eggs
¼ cup (½ stick) margarine

¼ teaspoon salt
2 teaspoons vanilla extract
½ cup unsweetened cocoa
   powder
Dry brown sugar substitute
   equal to ½ cup brown
   sugar

Place brown sugar and yeast in a mixer bowl. Mix lightly and add water. Let stand for 5 to 10 minutes, or until foamy. Add 1 cup of the flour and mix at medium speed (use a dough hook) for 4 minutes. Add eggs, margarine, salt, vanilla, remaining flour, cocoa, and dry brown sugar substitute. Mix at medium speed for 4 minutes. Spread dough evenly (it will be sticky) in a 9 × 5-inch loaf pan that has been sprayed with cooking spray or greased with margarine. Cover the pan with wax paper and a clean cloth, and let dough rise to the top of the pan.

Bake at 350°F for about 45 minutes, or until bread is firm and the bottom sounds hollow when thumped. Remove the pan to a wire rack, and after 10 to 15 minutes turn bread out onto the rack to cool to room temperature. Cut into 18 equal slices ½ inch wide.

Yield: 18 servings
Food exchanges per serving: 1 starch and 1 fat; or 1 carbohydrate
   choice
Sugar per serving: Negligible
Low-cholesterol diets: Omit eggs. Use ½ cup egg whites or liquid egg
   substitute.
Low-sodium diets: Omit salt. Use salt-free margarine.
Nutritive values per serving:

Calories: 97
CHO: 14 g
PRO: 3 g

FAT: 4 g
Na: 67 mg
Cholesterol: 30 g

Panettone

My husband's relatives used to send us panettone from Italy, and I never could duplicate the recipe until I started using bread flour and anise seed. Traditionally it is a round loaf, but I bake it in a rectangular loaf pan because it is easier for me to cut uniform portions that way.

1½ cups very hot water	2 teaspoons salt
¼ cup instant nonfat dry milk	2 large eggs
Dry sugar substitute equal to ½ cup sugar	⅓ cup (⅔ stick) margarine at room temperature
2 envelopes (2¼ teaspoons each) Rapid Rise active dry yeast	1 tablespoon anise seed
	¼ cup raisins
4¾ cups bread flour	¼ cup chopped candied fruit

Place water, dry milk, and sugar substitute in a mixer bowl. Mix lightly and cool to between 110° and 115°F. Add yeast, mix lightly, and let stand for 5 to 10 minutes. Add 2 cups of the flour and mix at medium speed (use a dough hook) for 4 minutes. Add salt, eggs, margarine, anise seed, raisins, candied fruit, and 2½ cups of the flour, and mix at medium speed for 2 to 3 minutes. Sprinkle remaining ¼ cup flour on a work surface and turn dough out onto flour. Knead 10 to 15 times, using as much of the flour as necessary to form a smooth, resilient dough. Form dough into a ball and place it in a bowl that has been sprayed with cooking spray or greased with margarine. Sprinkle flour left on the work surface evenly over dough, cover with a clean cloth, and let dough rise until doubled in volume.

Turn dough out onto a lightly floured surface, divide into two equal portions, and form each into a ball. Cover each with a clean cloth and let rest for 10 minutes. Form into loaves and place each loaf in a 9 × 5-inch loaf pan that has been sprayed with cooking spray or greased with margarine. Cover each with a clean cloth and let dough rise until doubled in volume.

Bake at 350°F for about 1 hour, or until loaves are golden brown and firm. Remove from pans and cool to room temperature. Cut each loaf into 18 equal slices ½ inch wide.

Yield: 36 (1-slice) servings
Food exchanges per serving: 1 starch; or 1 carbohydrate choice
Sugar per serving: None
Low-cholesterol diets: Omit eggs. Use ½ cup egg whites or liquid egg substitute.
Low-sodium diets: Omit salt. Use salt-free margarine.
Nutritive values per serving:

Calories: 89	FAT: 1 g
CHO: 15 g	Na: 145 mg
PRO: 2 g	Cholesterol: 10 mg

Light Bran Bread

1 cup All-Bran, Bran
   Buds, Fiber One, or
   100% Bran
1½ cups all-purpose flour
⅓ cup sugar
Dry sugar substitute equal to
   ¼ cup sugar (optional)
1 tablespoon baking powder

2 tablespoons instant nonfat dry
   milk
¼ teaspoon salt
1 cup water at room
   temperature
⅓ cup vegetable oil
1 large egg
1 teaspoon vanilla extract

Place cereal, flour, sugar, dry sugar substitute (if using), baking powder, dry milk, and salt in a mixer bowl; mix for 30 seconds at low speed to blend well. Stir water, oil, egg, and vanilla together with a fork to blend well, and add to flour mixture. Mix at medium speed only until flour is moistened. Spread dough evenly in a 9 × 5-inch loaf pan that has been sprayed with cooking spray or lined with aluminum foil.

Bake at 375°F for about 45 minutes, or until bread is lightly browned and a cake tester comes out clean from the center. Remove the pan to a wire rack for 10 minutes, and then turn loaf out onto the rack. Cut into 16 equal slices ½ inch wide. Serve warm.

Yield: 16 servings
Food exchanges per serving: 1 starch and 1 fat; or 1 carbohydrate
   choice
Sugar per serving: 1 teaspoon or 4 grams
Low-cholesterol diets: Omit egg. Use ¼ cup egg whites or liquid egg
   substitute.
Low-sodium diets: Omit salt. Use low-sodium baking powder.
Nutritive values per serving:

Calories: 115	FAT: 6 g
CHO: 16 g	Na: 143 mg
PRO: 2 g	Cholesterol: 17 mg

Raisin Bread

This recipe is based on the Irish barm brack, a special holiday bread.

1¼ cups very hot water
2 tablespoons instant nonfat dry milk
3 tablespoons sugar
Dry sugar substitute equal to ½ cup sugar
2 envelopes (2¼ teaspoons each) Rapid Rise active dry yeast

4¼ cups bread flour
2 teaspoons salt
¼ cup (½ stick) plus 1 tablespoon margarine
2 large eggs
½ cup raisins
¼ cup chopped fresh or dried orange peel
1 tablespoon sugar

Place water, dry milk, 2 tablespoons of the sugar, and dry sugar substitute in a mixer bowl. Mix lightly and cool to between 110° and 115°F. Add yeast, mix lightly, and let stand for 5 to 10 minutes, or until foamy. Add 2 cups of the flour and mix at medium speed (use a dough hook) for 4 minutes. Add salt, ¼ cup of the margarine, eggs, and another 2 cups of the flour, and mix for 4 minutes at medium speed. Add raisins and orange peel, and mix at low speed for 2 minutes.

Sprinkle remaining ¼ cup flour on a work surface and turn dough out onto it. Knead, using as much of the flour as necessary to form a smooth, resilient dough. Form dough into a ball and place in a bowl that has been well greased with margarine. Turn the ball over so the top will be greased, cover the bowl with a clean cloth, and let dough rise until doubled in volume.

Turn dough out onto a floured work surface. Knead lightly and divide into two equal parts. Form each into a ball and place on a lightly floured work surface. Cover and let rest for 10 minutes. Form each ball into a loaf and place each in a 9 × 5-inch loaf pan that has been sprayed with cooking spray or well greased with margarine. Cover each pan with a clean cloth and let dough rise at room temperature until doubled in volume.

Bake at 375°F for about 45 minutes, or until loaves are browned and firm. Turn loaves out onto a wire rack, rub the top and sides with 1 tablespoon margarine, and sprinkle with 1 tablespoon sugar. Cool to room temperature. Cut each loaf into 18 equal slices ½ inch wide.

Yield: 36 (1-slice) servings
Food exchanges per serving: 1 starch; or 1 carbohydrate choice
Sugar per serving: .3 teaspoon or 1 gram
Low-cholesterol diets: Omit eggs. Use ½ cup egg whites or liquid egg
  substitute.
Low-sodium diets: Omit salt. Use salt-free margarine.
Nutritive values per serving:

Calories: 83	FAT: 2 g
CHO: 14 g	Na: 143 mg
PRO: 2 g	Cholesterol: 15 mg

Raisin Bran Loaf

My sister used to take this bread back to Chicago with her after visiting me in Iowa. She said it stayed fresh and tasty, and reminded her of Iowa.

1 cup all-purpose flour
1½ cups All-Bran, Bran Buds, Fiber One, or 100% Bran
¼ cup sugar
¼ cup raisins
1 teaspoon baking soda
Dry sugar substitute equal to ¼ cup sugar
¼ teaspoon salt
1 cup water at room temperature
1 large egg
2 tablespoons molasses
1 tablespoon lemon juice
⅓ cup vegetable oil

Place flour, cereal, sugar, raisins, baking soda, dry sugar substitute, and salt in a mixer bowl; mix at low speed for 30 seconds to blend well. Stir water, egg, molasses, lemon juice, and oil together with a fork to blend well, and add to flour mixture. Mix at medium speed for 1 minute. Spread dough evenly in a 9 × 5-inch loaf pan that has been sprayed with cooking spray or greased with margarine.

Bake at 375°F for 45 minutes, or until bread pulls away from the sides of the pan and a cake tester comes out clean from the center. Remove the pan to a wire rack for 10 minutes, and then turn loaf out onto the rack to cool to room temperature. Cut into 16 equal slices ½ inch wide.

Yield: 16 (1-slice) servings
Food exchanges per serving: 1 starch and 1 fat; or 1 carbohydrate choice
Sugar per serving: 1.2 teaspoons or 5 grams
Low-cholesterol diets: Omit egg. Use ¼ cup egg whites or liquid egg substitute.
Low-sodium diets: Omit salt.
Nutritive values per serving:

Calories: 111
CHO: 17 g
PRO: 2 g
FAT: 5 g
Na: 152 mg
Cholesterol: 15 mg

Sweet Whole-Wheat Bread

I use this recipe when I want a sweet bread for breakfast or sandwiches but prefer not to use white bread. Be sure to use the bread flour. I'm depending on the extra gluten in the bread flour to make up for less gluten in whole-wheat flour and you won't get good results if you use all-purpose flour.

1 teaspoon sugar	1 teaspoon salt
1 envelope (2¼ teaspoons) Rapid Rise active dry yeast	¼ cup instant nonfat dry milk
¾ cup water at 110° to 115°F	1 teaspoon cinnamon (optional)
1¼ cups bread flour	2 large eggs at room temperature
1½ cups whole-wheat flour	
Dry brown sugar substitute equal to ½ cup brown sugar	2 tablespoons margarine at room temperature

Place sugar and yeast in a mixer bowl and mix lightly. Add water and let stand for 5 to 10 minutes, or until foamy. Add bread flour and mix at medium speed (use a dough hook) for 4 minutes. Stir together whole-wheat flour, dry brown sugar substitute, salt, dry milk, and cinnamon (if using), and blend well. Add eggs and margarine to bread flour mixture, and then add whole-wheat flour mixture. Mix at medium speed for 4 minutes, or until dough pulls away from the sides of the bowl. Turn dough out onto a floured work surface and knead a few times. Form dough into a ball and place it in a bowl that has been greased with margarine. Turn the ball over to grease the top. Cover the bowl with a clean cloth and let dough rise until doubled in volume.

Turn dough out onto a floured work surface, knead a few times, and form into a ball. Cover the ball and let it rest for 10 minutes. Form the ball into a loaf and place in a 9 × 5-inch loaf pan that has been sprayed with cooking spray or greased with margarine. Let dough rise until doubled in volume.

Bake at 350°F for about 1 hour, or until bread is browned and firm. Turn out onto a wire rack and cool to room temperature. Cut loaf into 18 equal slices ½ inch wide.

Yield: 18 (1-slice) servings
Food exchanges per serving: 1 starch; or 1 carbohydrate choice
Sugar per serving: Negligible
Low-cholesterol diets: Omit eggs. Use ½ cup egg whites or liquid egg substitute.
Low-sodium diets: Omit salt. Use salt-free margarine.
Nutritive values per serving:

Calories: 93	FAT: 2 g
CHO: 15 g	Na: 146 mg
PRO: 3 g	Cholesterol: 31 mg

CHAPTER 11

Fruits and Salads

FRUIT DESSERTS AND salads are typically quick and easy to make. They are also a great way to get in additional servings of fruits during the day. The light and refreshing taste of fruit can complement a hearty meal without leaving diners overly full.

Using fruits as a routine part of any meal can be a beneficial health habit. The sweetness found in fruit provides the finishing touch to almost any meal, and it curbs your appetite for sweets. Additionally, fruits are packed with vitamins and minerals, especially vitamins A and C, which help protect you from disease. Fresh fruits are a good source of fiber, which can help keep blood glucose levels in an acceptable range. Best yet, they come in a wide variety of great tastes.

As with all desserts, the quality of the ingredients you use affects your final product. This is particularly true when ending the meal with a fruit or a salad.

Here are some special things to remember when you are preparing fruits or salads:

1. To ensure delicious fruits and salads, select fruits that are top quality, free of bruises and spoilage, and fully ripe. The riper a fruit is, the more of a natural sweet flavor it will have. Overripe fruit, however, may give your fruit dish or salad an off flavor.

2. Handle fruit carefully. Dropping fruit can cause immediate bruising, a dark color, and a mushy texture.

3. Wash all fruit thoroughly to remove any dirt, waxes, or pesticides.

4. The nutrients in fruits tend to be more concentrated near the skin. Therefore, when peeling fruits, remove as little peel as possible, or incorporate the peel into the fruit dish or salad when appropriate.

5. When using apples, pears, and bananas in fruit dishes or salads, you can prevent them from turning brown, a process called enzymatic browning, by dipping them in either orange juice, pineapple juice, salt water, or Fruit Fresh.

6. When selecting canned fruits for fruit dishes or salads choose fruit packed in water or in natural juice. These methods of canning do not add additional sugar to the fruit.

7. Most frozen fruits come ready to eat or cook. When selecting frozen fruits, look for varieties without added sugar. Usually, it is best to thaw the fruit almost, but not completely; a few ice crystals should remain at serving time for frozen fruits to be at their best.

8. Gelatins can be used in fruit dishes and salads for added variety, color, and flavor, and they are easy to turn out right every time. Many companies make tasty sugar-free gelatins that don't add extra carbohydrates and sugars to your meals. And their refreshing flavors give them universal appeal to people of all ages. Fruit gelatin parfaits can be made quickly out of layers of flavored gelatin cubes and fruit with a dollop of whipped cream on top for a refreshing and healthy meal finale.

9. When preparing gelatins, make sure the gelatin is completely dissolved in the liquid before adding other ingredients or refrigerating.

10. Keeping gelatin covered in the refrigerator will prevent it from becoming tough and rubbery, drying out, and absorbing other food odors.

11. Molded gelatins and salads add a festive touch to any table. To successfully unmold a gelatin salad, lightly spray the mold with cooking spray before adding the gelatin or salad. Make sure the gelatin or salad is completely set before attempting to remove it from the mold. When you are ready to unmold the salad or gelatin, quickly dip the mold in and out of hot water up to ½ inch from the top of the mold. Place a serving dish on top of the mold; invert the mold and gently shake until the salad slips out. Lift off the mold and garnish. Return to the refrigerator if you are not planning on using within 15 minutes.

12. Only add canned pineapple to gelatin salads. Use of fresh pineapple in a gelatin salad will cause the gelatin to not set properly, as will fresh kiwifruit, figs, and papaya.

Cherry Cola Salad

This fruit or dessert salad may be topped with whipped topping or served on a lettuce leaf and garnished with 2 cherries or a quarter of a pineapple ring.

¾ cup water
⅓ cup sugar
20-ounce can light cherry pie
  filling
0.3-ounce package sugar-free
  cherry gelatin

20-ounce can crushed
  pineapple in juice or
  water (undrained)
1 tablespoon lemon juice
12 ounces cold diet cola
¼ cup chopped nuts (optional)

Combine water and sugar in a saucepan and bring to a boil. Add pie filling and return to a boil. Pour boiling mixture over gelatin, stirring to dissolve. Add pineapple with its liquid, lemon juice, cola, and nuts (if using). Pour into a 9 × 13-inch pan and chill. Cut three by five.

Yield: 15 servings
Food exchanges per serving: 1 fruit; or 1 carbohydrate choice
Sugar per serving: 3 teaspoons or 13 grams
Low-cholesterol diets: Recipe is suitable as written.
Low-sodium diets: Recipe is suitable as written. Use your own
  discretion for inclusion in your diet.
Nutritive values per serving:

Calories: 84
CHO: 15 g
PRO: 2 g

FAT: 1 g
Na: 115 mg
Cholesterol: 0

Lemony Fruit Sauce

Serve over cut-up fresh fruit, gingerbread, or Yellow Cake (page 64). The sauce can be refrigerated, tightly covered, for up to one week.

2 teaspoons (½ of a 0.3-ounce package) sugar-free lemon gelatin
1 cup boiling water

4 ounces frozen orange juice concentrate
8-ounce can chunk pineapple in juice or water (undrained)

In a 2½-quart bowl mix gelatin and boiling water. Stir in the orange juice and pineapple. Chill in the refrigerator until mixture is set. It will be soft, not firm. Makes 3 cups.

Yield: 24 (2-tablespoon) servings
Food exchanges: Free food
Sugar per serving: 0.5 teaspoon or 2 grams
Low-cholesterol diets: Recipe is suitable as written.
Low-sodium diets: Recipe is suitable as written.
Nutritive values per serving:

Calories: 11	FAT: 0
CHO: 3 g	Na: 9 mg
PRO: 0	Cholesterol: 0

Note: One serving of Lemony Fruit Sauce with ½ cup fruit provides 1½ fruit exchange or 18 grams of carbohydrate.

Mandarin Orange Fluff Salad

This easy fruit salad can be served as either a salad or a dessert. I like this salad because it is both delicious and simple to prepare. Reserve some of the mandarin orange segments for garnish if desired.

11-ounce can drained mandarin orange segments in juice or light syrup
1⅓ cups reduced-fat (2%) cottage cheese

1 cup light whipped topping
2 teaspoons (½ of a 0.3-ounce package) sugar-free orange gelatin

Drain mandarin oranges and reserve 2 tablespoons of the liquid. Place mandarin oranges, reserved liquid, cottage cheese, and whipped topping in a bowl. Sprinkle with sugar-free gelatin. Mix well. Cover and chill for at least 2 hours. Spoon into tulip or dessert cups.

Yield: 7 (½-cup) servings
Food exchanges per serving: ½ starch and ½ protein; or ½ carbohydrate choice
Sugar per serving: 1.2 teaspoons or 5 grams
Low-cholesterol diets: Recipe is suitable as written.
Low-sodium diets: Rinse cottage cheese. Use your own discretion for inclusion in your diet.
Nutritive values per serving:

Calories: 96
CHO: 9 g
PRO: 6 g

FAT: 3 g
Na: 192 mg
Cholesterol: 3 mg

Triple Lemon Salad

2 teaspoons (½ of a 0.3-ounce package) sugar-free lemon gelatin
½ cup boiling water
3 tablespoons chilled Diet Mountain Dew

¼ cup miniature marshmallows
½ cup canned lemon pie filling
¼ cup light whipped topping
Lemon twists for garnish

Dissolve gelatin in boiling water in a medium bowl. Stir in Mountain Dew. Chill mixture until almost set. Fold in the marshmallows, pie filling, and whipped topping. Mix well and chill until set. Serve in tulip cups and garnish with a lemon twist.

Yield: 6 (½-cup) servings
Food exchanges per serving: 1 starch; or 1 carbohydrate choice
Sugar per serving: 3.8 teaspoons or 16 grams
Low-cholesterol diets: Recipe is suitable as written.
Low-sodium diets: Recipe is suitable as written.
Nutritive values per serving:

Calories: 100	FAT: 2 g
CHO: 19 g	Na: 39 mg
PRO: 2 g	Cholesterol: 31 mg

Variation: For a dish lower in calories and carbohydrates, use ½ cup Lemon Cream Pudding (page 186) in place of the lemon pie filling.

Food exchanges per serving: ½ starch; or ½ carbohydrate choice
Sugar per serving: 1.4 teaspoons or 6 grams
Nutritive values per serving:

Calories: 39	FAT: 1 g
CHO: 7 g	Na: 29 mg
PRO: 1 g	Cholesterol: 11 mg

Pistachio Salad

A perfect quick and easy salad or dessert for St. Patrick's Day or anytime you want to add color and the nutty taste of pistachios to your meal. This salad can be put together in less than 5 minutes.

1⅓ cups reduced-fat (2%)
cottage cheese
8-ounce can crushed pineapple
in water or juice
(undrained)

¼ teaspoon vanilla extract
1 cup light whipped topping
7 teaspoons (½ of a 1-ounce
package) sugar-free pistachio
instant pudding

Combine cottage cheese, pineapple with its liquid, vanilla, and whipped topping in a bowl. Sprinkle pistachio pudding over all. Mix well. Cover and chill for at least 2 hours. Spoon into tulip or dessert cups.

Yield: 7 (½-cup) servings
Food exchanges per serving: 1 starch and ½ protein; or 1
carbohydrate choice
Sugar per serving: 1.7 teaspoons or 6.9 grams
Low-cholesterol diets: Recipe is suitable as written.
Low-sodium diets: Rinse cottage cheese. Use your own discretion for inclusion in your diet.
Nutritive values per serving:

Calories: 110
CHO: 13 g
PRO: 6 g

FAT: 3 g
Na: 273 mg
Cholesterol: 3 mg

Quick Fruit Salad

8-ounce crushed canned
    pineapple in juice or water
    (undrained)
½ teaspoon sugar
2 teaspoons (½ of a 0.3-ounce
    package) sugar-free orange
    gelatin
Dry sugar substitute equal to
    1 teaspoon sugar

1 cup buttermilk
1 cup light whipped
    topping
2 cups fresh fruit or drained
    canned fruit, packed in juice
    or water
2 tablespoons chopped walnuts
    (optional)

In a medium saucepan, mix the crushed pineapple (with its liquid) and sugar. Bring mixture to a boil and boil for 1 minute. Remove from heat and add gelatin and sugar substitute. Mix until dissolved.

Cool mixture until it is syrupy. Add buttermilk and whipped topping. Mix thoroughly. Fold in fruit and nuts (if using). Chill until mixture is set.

Yield: 6 (½-cup) servings
Food exchanges per serving: 2 fruit; or 1½ carbohydrate choices
Sugar per serving: 2.9 teaspoons or 12 grams
Low-cholesterol diets: Recipe is suitable as written.
Low-sodium diets: Recipe is suitable as written. Use your own
    discretion for inclusion in your diet.
Nutritive values per serving:

Calories: 132	FAT: 3 g
CHO: 14 g	Na: 67 mg
PRO: 2 g	Cholesterol: 1 mg

Red-Hot Cinnamon Salad

This salad adds color to any meal, but it is especially tasty with poultry. Whipped topping may be used as a garnish.

¼ cup Red-Hot Cinnamon
  candies
2 cups boiling water
2 (0.3-ounce) packages sugar-
  free cherry or strawberry

gelatin
2 cups strained unsweetened
  applesauce

In a 2½-quart glass bowl dissolve candies in boiling water. Add gelatin and mix until it is dissolved. Fold in applesauce until blended.

Cover and refrigerate for 3 hours, or until set.

Note: Gelatin mixture can be poured into a heart-shaped mold that has been sprayed with cooking spray. Chill for at least 3 hours. Unmold and garnish.

Yield: 8 (½-cup) servings
Food exchanges per serving: 1 starch; or 1 carbohydrate choice
Sugar per serving: 1.5 teaspoons or 6.25 grams
Low-cholesterol diets: Recipe is suitable as written.
Low-sodium diets: Recipe is suitable as written.
Nutritive values per serving:

Calories: 80	FAT: 0
CHO: 18 g	Na: 55 mg
PRO: 1 g	Cholesterol: 0

Rhubarb Salad

It's best to make this in the spring when fresh rhubarb is available.

1½ cups boiling water
1½ cups diced fresh or frozen
   rhubarb
3 tablespoons sugar
1 (0.6-ounce) package or
  2 (0.3-ounce) packages
  sugar-free raspberry or
  cherry gelatin

1 cup cold water
1½ tablespoons lemon juice
10-ounce can (1¼ cups)
  crushed pineapple
  (drained)
⅓ cup chopped celery
¼ cup chopped pecans or
  walnuts (optional)

In a saucepan, bring boiling water, rhubarb, and sugar to a boil. Cook rhubarb over medium heat until it is soft. Remove from heat and add gelatin. Mix until dissolved. Add cold water and lemon juice. Pour into a bowl and chill until mixture begins to set, about 45 minutes. Add pineapple, celery, and nuts (if using). Pour into an 8-inch square pan. Chill until set. Cut three by three.

Yield: 9 servings
Food exchanges per serving: 1 fruit; or ½ carbohydrate choice
Sugar per serving: 1.4 teaspoons or 6 grams
Low-cholesterol diets: Recipe is suitable as written.
Low-sodium diets: Recipe is suitable at your discretion.
Nutritive values per serving:

Calories: 89
CHO: 7 g
PRO: 5 g

FAT: 3 g
  (0 if nuts are omitted)
Na: 230 mg
Cholesterol: 0

Rosy Rhubarb-Strawberry Salad

Fresh strawberries and rhubarb combine to make this beautiful spring salad a tangy delight either with or at the end of a meal.

4 cups diced rhubarb
1¾ cups water
¼ cup sugar
Dry sugar substitute equal to
  ¼ cup sugar

2 (1-ounce) packages sugar-free
  strawberry gelatin
¾ cup orange juice
1 teaspoon grated orange rind
1 cup sliced strawberries

Combine rhubarb, water, and sugar in a saucepan. Cook over medium heat until the rhubarb is tender. Remove from heat. Add gelatin and dry sugar substitute. Stir until the gelatin is completely dissolved. Add the orange juice and orange rind. Mix well.

Chill until syrupy, about 30 minutes. Add strawberries. Pour into a 1½-quart serving bowl or a lightly oiled 6-cup mold. Chill until firm and set.

Yield: 8 (¾-cup) servings
Food exchanges per serving: 1 fruit; or 1 carbohydrate choice
Sugar per serving: 2.6 teaspoons or 11 grams
Low-cholesterol diets: Recipe is suitable as written.
Low-sodium diets: Recipe is suitable as written. Use your own
  discretion for inclusion in your diet.
Nutritive values per serving:

Calories: 77
CHO: 13 g
PRO: 5 g

FAT: 0
Na: 160 mg
Cholesterol: 0

Sparkling Melon Salad

This refreshing spring or summer salad turns fruit easily into a dessert.

1 cup plus 2 tablespoons apple juice
0.3-ounce package sugar-free mandarin orange gelatin

¾ cup cold club soda
¾ cup each cantaloupe and honeydew melon cubes

In a saucepan, bring apple juice to a boil. Dissolve gelatin completely in the boiling apple juice. Stir in club soda. Refrigerate about 45 minutes, or until slightly thickened and cool.

Stir in 1 cup of the melon cubes. Spoon into a 3- to 4-cup mold that has been lightly sprayed with cooking spray. Refrigerate 4 hours or until firm. Unmold. Garnish with remaining melon cubes. If desired, salad can be set in a serving bowl.

Variation: Sparkling Strawberry Salad: Substitute 1½ cups sliced fresh strawberries for the melon and sugar-free strawberry gelatin for the mandarin orange gelatin.

Yield: 6 (½-cup) servings
Food exchanges per serving: 1 fruit; or 1 carbohydrate choice
Sugar per serving: 2 teaspoons or 9 grams
Low-cholesterol diets: Recipe is suitable as written.
Low-sodium diets: Recipe is suitable as written.
Nutritive values per serving:

Calories: 50
CHO: 11 g
PRO: 2 g
FAT: 0
Na: 80 mg
Cholesterol: 0

Spiced Fruit

Spiced fruit is a nice change of pace from traditional fruit salads. Served chilled, it complements a cold sandwich or warm pork roast on an autumn day.

15.25-ounce can pears, in juice or water

15.25-ounce can peaches, in juice or water

20-ounce can pineapple chunks or tidbits, in juice

2 teaspoons whole cloves

1/4 teaspoon nutmeg

1 cinnamon stick, broken into several pieces

2 oranges, peeled and segmented

Drain fruits, reserving the pear juice separately. Cut up pears and peaches into bite-size pieces. Place pear juice, cloves, nutmeg, and cinnamon in a large saucepan and bring to a boil. Reduce heat and simmer for 5 minutes. Add fruits (except oranges) to simmering liquid and return to a boil. Remove from heat and discard cloves and cinnamon pieces. Cool slightly. Halve orange segments crosswise and stir into fruit mixture.

Refrigerate for at least 6 to 8 hours before serving, to blend flavors.

Yield: 10 (1/2-cup) servings
Food exchanges per serving: 1 fruit; or 1 carbohydrate choice
Sugar per serving: 3.8 teaspoons or 16 grams
Low-cholesterol diets: Recipe is suitable as written.
Low-sodium diets: Recipe is suitable as written.
Nutritive values per serving:

Calories: 76
CHO: 20 g
PRO: 1 g

FAT: 0
Na: 5 mg
Cholesterol: 0

Hot Fruit Compote

2 apples, such as McIntosh, Cortland, or Jonathan, peeled and thinly sliced
15.25-ounce can peach slices in juice or water, drained
15.25-ounce can apricot halves in juice or water, drained
15.25-ounce can pear halves in juice or water, drained
1/4 cup maraschino cherries (optional)

1/2 cup orange juice
1/4 cup packed brown sugar
1/2 teaspoon ground cinnamon
1/4 teaspoon nutmeg
4 whole cloves
1/8 teaspoon ground mace (optional)
1/8 teaspoon salt

In a 2-1/2-quart baking dish, combine the apples, peaches, apricots, pears, and cherries (if using); set aside.

In a small saucepan, combine the remaining ingredients and bring to a boil over medium heat; pour over fruit. Bake, uncovered, at 350°F for 25 to 30 minutes or until bubbly. Discard cloves. Serve warm.

Yield: 14 (1/2-cup) servings
Food exchanges per serving: 1 fruit; or 1 carbohydrate choice
Sugar per serving: 4 teaspoons or 17 grams
Low-cholesterol diets: Recipe is suitable as written.
Low-sodium diets: Recipe is suitable as written.
Nutritive values per serving:

Calories: 75   FAT: 0
CHO: 19 g   Na: 29 mg
PRO: 1 g   Cholesterol: 0

CHAPTER 12

$\mathcal{D}$essers

THROUGHOUT THIS BOOK, we have given you a multitude of ideas and recipes for cakes, puddings, pies, bars, salads, fruits, and cookies. This final chapter contains recipes that do not fit into any of the previous categories, but are traditionally known as desserts.

Whether it is simple or elegant, a dessert should end the meal on an impressive note. The primary purpose of serving a dessert is to complement and finish the meal in a way that is satisfying to the diner, without being overly filling. Desserts can also give you that final chance to fill the day's quota for milk, fruit, or bread. When planning the menu, you may want to choose a dessert that balances the entrée. If the meal has included a hearty entrée, a light dessert may be in order. However, a more filling dessert can be a nice contrast to a lighter entrée.

Here are some special ideas to remember when you are preparing or serving desserts:

1. Keep in mind that the temperature of the dessert is important. Some desserts are best served warm, like cobblers and crisps. Others, like gelatin desserts, are best served chilled. Frozen desserts are best if allowed to stand at room temperature for a few minutes before serving.

2. For desserts that have reduced-sugar or lower-sugar ingredients, you can enhance the flavor and sweetness by adding very small amounts of sugar, chocolate curls, or slices of fresh fruit to the finished product. For example, a sprinkle of brown sugar over the top of an

apple crisp can enhance the sweetness or a strawberry partially dipped in chocolate can complement an unfrosted piece of angel food cake.

3. Many times a smaller portion of a regular dessert can provide as much satisfaction as a larger portion when it is eaten in a relaxing environment at a slow pace. Many people find that when they allow themselves the experience of eating slowly and savoring their food it takes less of an item to be satisfying.

4. Most of all remember that all foods can fit into your meal plan; this includes luscious, tantalizing desserts. Trust that you can use these foods and monitor your own blood glucose response to various after-meal favorites. Bon appétit!

Creamy Raspberry Dessert

My mother-in-law, Jeanne Blocker, of Waukon, Iowa, makes this light and creamy summer sensation that brings fruit to the dessert table.

Graham Cracker–Pretzel Crust

8 (2¼-inch) graham cracker squares
1 cup pretzels

⅓ cup reduced-fat margarine, melted

Filling

0.3-ounce package sugar-free raspberry gelatin
½ cup boiling water
1¼ cups sugar-free frozen vanilla yogurt
1½ cups fresh or frozen unsweetened raspberries (drained if frozen)

¼ cup lime juice
8-ounce carton (2 cups) whipped topping
Lime slices, additional raspberries, and whipped topping for garnish (optional)

Finely crush the graham crackers and pretzels with a rolling pin or in a blender or food processor. Transfer mixture to a 7 × 11-inch glass baking dish. Add the margarine and mix together. Pat the mixture evenly into the bottom of the dish. Bake at 350°F for 5 to 10 minutes, or until lightly browned. Cool before filling.

Dissolve gelatin in boiling water in a mixing bowl. Stir in frozen yogurt until melted. Add the raspberries and lime juice. Fold in whipped topping. Spoon into crust.

Refrigerate for 3 hours or until firm. Cut into 12 equal pieces. Garnish with lime slices, raspberries, and whipped topping as desired.

Yield: 12 servings
Food exchanges per serving: 1 starch, ½ fruit, and 1 fat; or 1 carbohydrate choice
Sugar per serving: 1.7 teaspoons or 7 grams
Low-cholesterol diets: Recipe is suitable as written. May want to use light or fat-free whipped topping.
Low-sodium diets: Use unsalted pretzels. Use your own discretion for inclusion in your diet.
Nutritive values per serving:

Calories: 145	FAT: 6 g
CHO: 18g	Na: 330 mg
PRO: 6 g	Cholesterol: 0

Cream Puff Dessert

My sister, Evie Milbrandt, makes this dessert for special occasions. I made a lower-sugar version for this book. If you enjoy cream puffs, you'll like this easy-to-make dessert, which is similar to a giant cream puff.

Fran's Cream Puffs (page 176)

Filling

1-ounce package reduced-calorie, sugar-free instant vanilla or chocolate pudding

8-ounce package light cream cheese

1½ cups fat-free milk

Topping

1 cup light whipped topping

2 tablespoons Hershey's chocolate syrup

Make cream puff batter according to recipe directions. Spread batter in a lightly greased 8-inch square pan. Bake at 400°F for 30 minutes. Cool puff shell.

Cut in half horizontally and add filling. Spread with whipped topping and drizzle with chocolate syrup. Refrigerate until serving. Cut two by four.

Yield: 8 servings
Food exchanges: 1 starch and 1½ fat; or 1½ carbohydrate choices
Sugar per serving: 1.2 teaspoons or 5 grams
Low-cholesterol diets: Liquid egg substitutes do not work well in the recipe for Fran's Cream Puffs. Use your own discretion for inclusion in your diet.
Low-sodium diets: Use your own discretion for inclusion in your diet.
Nutritive values per serving:

Calories: 163   FAT: 7 g
CHO: 23 g   Na: 204 mg
PRO: 5 g   Cholesterol: 86 mg

Fluffy Strawberry Gelatin Dessert

This refreshing dessert is always a hit with family and friends, especially in the early summer when strawberries are at their best.

Crust

1 cup graham cracker crumbs (about 20 2¼-inch squares)
1 teaspoon cinnamon

Dry sugar substitute equal to 1 tablespoon sugar
3 tablespoons margarine, melted

Filling

2 cups sliced fresh strawberries
1 tablespoon sugar
0.3-ounce package sugar-free strawberry gelatin
½ cup boiling water

4 cups miniature marshmallows
½ cup fat-free milk
½ teaspoon vanilla extract
8-ounce carton (2 cups) reduced-fat whipped topping

For crust: In a bowl, combine cracker crumbs, cinnamon, dry sugar substitute, and margarine. Press into a 9 × 13-inch baking dish that has been sprayed with cooking spray. Bake at 350°F for 8 to 10 minutes or until golden brown. Cool on a wire rack.

For filling: Combine strawberries and sugar in a small bowl; let stand for 20 minutes. In another bowl, dissolve gelatin in boiling water. Cool gelatin until it begins to set. Drain berries, reserving the juice. To the juice add enough water to measure 1 cup. Stir berries and juice mixture into gelatin. Refrigerate until syrupy.

Meanwhile, combine marshmallows and milk in a saucepan. Cook and stir over low heat until blended and smooth. Stir in vanilla. Cool to room temperature, about 15 minutes. Fold in whipped topping, then gelatin mixture. Pour into the prepared crust. Refrigerate for 4 hours, or until firm. Cut three by five.

Note: Frozen strawberries can be substituted if fresh are not available.

Yield: 15 servings

Food exchanges per serving: 1½ starch; or 2 carbohydrate choices

Sugar per serving: 3.4 teaspoons or 14 grams

Low-cholesterol diets: Recipe is suitable as written.

Low-sodium diets: Use salt-free margarine. Use your own discretion for inclusion in your diet.

Nutritive values per serving:

Calories: 127	FAT: 4 g
CHO: 25 g	Na: 87 mg
PRO: 2 g	Cholesterol: 0

Lemon Dessert

My aunt Anita Herold would bring this dessert to holiday family gatherings. It is so light and refreshing and a perfect complement to calorie-laden holiday meals.

Crust

10 (2¼-inch) graham cracker squares
Dry sugar substitute equivalent to 1½ teaspoons

1½ tablespoons margarine, melted

Filling

¼ cup sugar
3 tablespoons Splenda or a dry sugar substitute equivalent to ⅓ cup, suitable for use in cooking
1 large egg, beaten

8-ounce can crushed pineapple in water or juice pack (undrained)
0.3-ounce package sugar-free lemon gelatin
⅔ cup fat-free evaporated milk, chilled

For crust: Crush graham crackers until very fine. Stir in dry sugar substitute. Add melted margarine and mix. Reserve 2 tablespoons of the mixture. Pat remaining mixture into the bottom of an 8-inch square pan. Bake at 350°F for 5 to 10 minutes in oven. Cool before filling.

For filling: Bring sugar, sugar substitute, egg, and pineapple to a boil in a saucepan over medium heat and boil for 2 minutes. Stir in gelatin and mix well. Set aside to cool completely.

Whip the chilled evaporated milk until soft peaks form. (Be sure the milk, beaters, and bowl are very cold.) Fold in the pineapple mixture. Pour over the graham cracker crust. Sprinkle reserved crumbs on top. Refrigerate until set. Cut two by four.

Yield: 8 servings
Food exchanges per serving: 1 starch and ½ fat; or 1 carbohydrate choice
Sugar per serving: 3 teaspoons or 12 grams
Low-cholesterol diets: Omit egg. Use ¼ cup egg whites or liquid egg substitute.
Low-sodium diets: Recipe is suitable as written. Use your own discretion for inclusion in your diet.
Nutritive values per serving:

Calories: 103	FAT: 3 g
CHO: 16 g	Na: 103 mg
PRO: 2 g	Cholesterol: 14 mg

Double Chocolate and Peanut Butter Frozen Delight

If you like Snicker's candy bars, then this dessert will tantalize your taste buds. Preparation time is less than 5 minutes. Tightly covered, this dessert will keep in the freezer for a week.

1 pint (2 cups) sugar-free, low-fat chocolate ice cream or frozen low-fat yogurt
1 cup light whipped topping
¼ cup crunchy peanut butter
1 teaspoon vanilla extract

1-ounce package reduced-calorie, sugar-free white chocolate or vanilla pudding (not instant)
Hershey's chocolate syrup, for decoration

Place all ingredients except chocolate syrup into a mixer bowl and beat with an electric mixer until smooth and well blended. Pour the mixture into an 8-inch square pan. Drizzle a small amount of chocolate syrup decoratively on top of the ice cream mixture. Cover with plastic wrap and freeze until firm, about 4 hours or overnight. Cut the dessert into 8 equal servings.

Note: If you cannot find sugar-free chocolate ice cream or frozen yogurt, vanilla also works well.

Yield: 8 servings
Food exchanges per serving: 1 starch and 1 fat; or 1 carbohydrate choice
Sugar per serving: 1 teaspoon or 4 grams
Low-cholesterol diets: Recipe is suitable as written.
Low-sodium diets: Use low-salt peanut butter.
Nutritive values per serving:

Calories: 119
CHO: 15 g
PRO: 4 g
FAT: 6 g
Na: 170 mg
Cholesterol: 0

Apple Crisp

½ cup quick-cooking rolled oats
¼ cup packed brown sugar
Brown sugar substitute equal to
    1½ tablespoons
¼ cup all-purpose flour
½ teaspoon ground cinnamon
⅛ teaspoon salt
3 tablespoons butter or
    margarine
1 teaspoon vanilla extract
2 pounds apples (about 6
    medium)
1 tablespoon granulated sugar
Whipped topping (optional)

Combine oats, brown sugar, brown sugar substitute, flour, cinnamon, and salt. Cut in butter until mixture resembles coarse crumbs; stir in vanilla. Set aside.

Peel, core, and slice apples to make 5 to 6 cups. Place fruit in a 12 × 8-inch baking dish. Sprinkle with granulated sugar. Sprinkle crumb mixture over top.

Bake at 350°F for 40 to 45 minutes. Serve with whipped topping if desired (whipped topping is not included in the nutrient analysis). Cut five by two.

Yield: 10 servings
Food exchanges per serving: 1½ starch; or 1½ carbohydrate choices
Sugar per serving: 3.8 teaspoons or 16 grams
Low-cholesterol diets: Recipe is suitable as written.
Low-sodium diets: Omit salt. Use salt-free butter or margarine.
Nutritive values per serving:

Calories: 126   FAT: 4 g
CHO: 23 g   Na: 43 mg
PRO: 1 g   Cholesterol: 0

Variation: Peach Crisp: Substitute 2½ pounds (about 10) peaches for the apples.

Yield: 10 servings
Food exchanges per serving: 1½ starch; or 1½ carbohydrate choice
Sugar per serving: 3.6 teaspoons or 15 grams
Low-cholesterol diets: Recipe is suitable as written.
Low-sodium diets: Omit salt. Use salt-free butter or margarine.
Nutritive values per serving:

Calories: 121   FAT: 4 g
CHO: 22 g   Na: 43 mg
PRO: 2 g   Cholesterol: 0

Sour Cream Apple Dessert

This apple dessert is as tasty as apple pie without the extra calories.

¼ cup sugar
3 tablespoons all-purpose flour
Dry sugar substitute equal to 3 tablespoons sugar
¼ teaspoon nutmeg
¼ teaspoon cinnamon
⅛ teaspoon salt
8 ounces reduced-fat sour cream
2 large eggs, lightly beaten
1 teaspoon vanilla extract
3½ cups peeled, diced cooking apples, such as McIntosh or Cortland

Mix together sugar, flour, dry sugar substitute, nutmeg, cinnamon, and salt. Beat in sour cream, eggs, and vanilla. Stir apples into batter. Divide mixture into 7 (6-ounce) ramekins or custard cups.

Bake at 450°F for 15 minutes. Lower heat to 325°F and bake until tops are well browned and filling is set, 30 to 45 minutes. Cool to room temperature and chill.

Yield: 7 servings
Food exchanges per serving: 1 fruit and ½ starch; or 1 carbohydrate choice
Sugar per serving: 3.2 teaspoons or 13 grams
Low-cholesterol diets: Omit eggs. Use ½ cup liquid egg substitute.
Low-sodium diets: Omit salt.
Nutritive values per serving:

Calories: 123	FAT: 4 g
CHO: 20 g	Na: 80 mg
PRO: 3 g	Cholesterol: 74 mg

Chocolate-Filled Tortilla Cups

Kids like these dessert cups after school, at birthday parties, or at the end of a meal.

2 teaspoons sugar
Dry sugar substitute equal to
  1 teaspoon sugar

½ teaspoon ground
  cinnamon
4 (6-inch) flour tortillas

Filling

¼ cup reduced-fat cream
  cheese at room
  temperature
4 tablespoons cold fat-free
  milk
½ teaspoon vanilla
  extract

4 teaspoons (¼ of a 1-ounce
  package) reduced-calorie,
  sugar-free instant white
  chocolate pudding mix
½ cup light whipped
  topping
1 tablespoon chocolate syrup

In a small bowl, combine sugar, dry sugar substitute, and cinnamon. Coat one side of each tortilla with cooking spray; sprinkle with cinnamon sugar. Turn tortillas over; repeat on the other sides. Cut each tortilla into 4 wedges. For each dessert cup, place round edge of one tortilla wedge in the bottom of a muffin cup, shaping sides to fit cup. Place a second tortilla wedge in muffin cup, allowing bottom and sides to overlap. Bake at 350°F for 10 minutes, or until crisp and lightly browned. Cool completely in pan. Makes 8 cups.

Meanwhile, for filling, beat cream cheese in a bowl until smooth. In another bowl, beat milk, vanilla, and pudding mix on low speed for 2 minutes. Beat in cream cheese on low until smooth. Fold in whipped topping. Cover and refrigerate for 1 hour.

Carefully remove cups from pan. Pipe or spoon about 1½ tablespoons filling (level no. 40 dipper) into each cup. Drizzle with chocolate syrup. Refrigerate for 5 to 10 minutes or until chocolate is set. Store in the refrigerator.

Yield: 8 servings

Food exchanges per serving: 1 starch and ½ fat; or 1 carbohydrate
  choice

Sugar per serving: .5 teaspoon or 2 grams

Low-cholesterol diets: Recipe is suitable as written. May use fat-free
  cream cheese and fat-free whipped topping if desired.

Low-sodium diets: Recipe is suitable as written. Use your own
  discretion for including in your diet.

Nutritive values per serving:

Calories: 90	FAT: 3 g
CHO: 14 g	Na: 97 mg
PRO: 3 g	Cholesterol: 4 mg

Index

About the Authors

Mabel Cavaiani, R.D., wrote twelve other cookbooks, among them *The High Fiber Cookbook for Diabetics* (Perigee, 1987) and was the author of many magazine articles. She lived most of her working life in Chicago, where she spent some time in restaurant management and was the army representative on the Armed Forces Recipe Service for several years. Also, she lived in Wadena, Iowa, where she was a dietary consultant in nursing homes. She was involved in developing and publishing recipes for modified diets up until her death.

Anne Blocker, R.D./L.D., has a degree in Community-Medical Dietetics and over fifteen years of experience in medical nutrition therapy. Currently she is the Director of Nutrition Services at Veterans Memorial Hospital in Waukon, Iowa, where she delivers both in- and outpatient nutrition care. She is currently a member of the hospital's diabetes self-management education team. In addition, she works as a nutrition therapist, helping persons with eating disorders normalize their relationships with food.

She has previously authored or co-authored six books and has contributed articles to magazines and newspapers. She speaks regularly on nutrition, wellness, and health.